# ESSENTIAL READINGS IN MEDICINE AND RELIGION

# ESSENTIAL READINGS IN MEDICINE AND RELIGION

*Gary B. Ferngren and Ekaterina N. Lomperis*

Johns Hopkins University Press

*Baltimore*

Johns Hopkins University Press
2715 North Charles Street
Baltimore, Maryland 21218-4363
www.press.jhu.edu


Library of Congress Cataloging-in-Publication Data

Names: Ferngren, Gary B., editor. | Lomperis, Ekaterina N., 1983– editor. |
Complemented by (work): Ferngren, Gary B. Medicine and religion.
Title: Essential readings in Medicine and religion / [edited by] Gary B. Ferngren
and Ekaterina N. Lomperis.
Description: Baltimore : Johns Hopkins University Press, 2017. | Complemented
by: Medicine and religion / Gary B. Ferngren. [2014]. | Includes bibliographical
references and index.
Identifiers: LCCN 2016044785| ISBN 9781421422909 (pbk. : alk. paper) |
ISBN 1421422905 (pbk. : alk. paper) | ISBN 9781421422916 (electronic) |
ISBN 1421422913 (electronic)
Subjects: LCSH: Medicine—Religious aspects. | MESH: Religion and Medicine |
History of Medicine | Collected Works
Classification: LCC BL65.M4 E895 2017 | NLM BL 65.M4 | DDC 201/.661—dc23
LC record available at https://lccn.loc.gov/2016044785

A catalog record for this book is available from the British Library.

*Special discounts are available for bulk purchases of this book.*
*For more information, please contact Special Sales at 410-516-6936 or*
*specialsales@press.jhu.edu.*

*To my husband and son*

—EKATERINA LOMPERIS

*To my grandchildren,*
*James, Julian, Lexi, Max, Claire, Sophia, Amikha, Lilah,*
*Cole, Alexander, Annalise, Andrew*

—GARY FERNGREN

# CONTENTS

# PREFACE

This book is intended as a companion volume to *Medicine and Religion: A Historical Introduction* (Johns Hopkins University Press, 2014), which traces the history of the relationship of medicine to religion from the earliest ancient Near Eastern societies to the twenty-first century. The purpose of this volume is to provide an extensive selection of texts that expand and illustrate the narrative of the earlier book. Because the earlier volume covers a broad chronological expanse, it proved impossible to incorporate more than a few primary texts for each historical era. Our intention here is to enhance *Medicine and Religion*'s themes with a collection of primary sources that range in length from a few lines to several pages.

Our division of labor reflects our respective specialties in the history of medicine and religion. Gary Ferngren has assembled the texts and provided the commentary for chapters 1, 2, 3, and 4 (the ancient world), while Ekaterina Lomperis has selected the texts and written the commentary for chapters 5, 7, and 8 (the medieval and modern periods). She has also adapted two of the published translations (Burton's *Anatomy of Melancholy* and Ignatius of Loyola's *Spiritual Exercises*). Mujeeb Khan, a specialist in Islamic medicine and religion, has chosen and edited the texts for chapter 6 (Islam); he offers here three new translations of texts not previously available in English [6.4, 6.5, 6.7].

This volume supplies a collection of texts and places them in their respective contexts in order to specifically address the historical relationships between medicine and religion. Several other collections feature sources for the history of medicine. But thus far there has not appeared an educational volume focusing on the intersection of medicine and religion that covers the entire chronological sweep from ancient to modern. We hope that our volume proves to be a useful introduction for students interested in this growing field. We are happy to acknowledge that we have been greatly helped by earlier collections of texts, from which we have drawn freely. Knowledgeable readers will observe that we have omitted many texts that might have been profitably included had greater space been available.

This book is not a history of either medicine or religion, but of the intersection of the two. The fact that we include few descriptions of solely natural or empirical medicine might give the impression that traditional cultures relied on religious healing to the exclusion of empirical therapy. That is not true, but, as our sources indicate, religion played many roles beyond that of healing, which medicine alone could not provide.

The eight chapters in this volume parallel the eight chapters in *Medicine and Religion: A Historical Introduction*. Each chapter begins with a brief introduction that provides a basic historical context for the intersection of medicine and religion in the period covered. A more detailed medical-historical background is, of course, provided by the earlier book. The texts are numbered sequentially within each chapter and preceded by a short paragraph that contextualizes the author and subject. Throughout the book, square-bracketed numbers point readers to specific texts. While we have not keyed each text to the subjects treated in *Medicine and Religion*, the parallel organization of the chapters will permit readers to connect the material here to the appropriate historical narrative given there. All of the excerpts have been reproduced as they were published in the cited sources, including parenthetical comments and square-bracketed insertions from the original editors; ellipses indicate where material has been omitted because of space considerations. In a few cases, the authors of this book inserted some words of clarification or slightly modified older translations (both changes are indicated by curly brackets). The bibliography gives full citations for the sources from which we have taken the texts included in this volume.

# ACKNOWLEDGMENTS

We are grateful for the cooperation that has marked every phase of our collaborative work, during which each other's expertise, intellectual openness, and friendship have meant much to both of us.

Ekaterina Lomperis is grateful for the erudition and expertise of the colleagues who took the time to read her chapters, in particular Michelle Harrington, Daniel Kim, Mark Lambert, and Father John Schroedel. Her work owes a great deal to their feedback. Special thanks are owed to her doctoral advisor, Susan E. Schreiner, who helped her more fully to appreciate the complexities of the histories of both religion and medicine. The Johns Hopkins University Press team, in particular editor Jacqueline Wehmueller, were outstanding in navigating the manuscript's preparation. Ekaterina's mother and grandmother, although many miles away, supplied warm encouragement and inspiration from across the ocean. Most of all, Ekaterina would like to thank her husband, without whose unlimited patience, unconditional love, and self-sacrificial support at every stage of the manuscript preparation this book would not have happened.

Gary Ferngren expresses his warm appreciation for all who aided in this project, especially his personal assistant, Joy McMurchy, and his editorial assistant, Celia Funk. Their dedication, expertise, and care at every stage of the manuscript's preparation lightened his load considerably and made possible the completion of the book in a timely manner. Thanks to Mark Geller, who made suggestions for chapter 1; Ildiko Csepregi, who read chapters 2, 3, and 4; Jonathan Katz and Glen Cooper, who read chapter 6; and the anonymous readers of the press. As always, our editor, Jackie Wehmueller, and her staff at Johns Hopkins University Press have provided support and encouragement at every stage.

We also express our appreciation to the School of History, Philosophy, and Religion and to the Center for the Humanities and the Office of Research at Oregon State University, as well as to Johns Hopkins University Press, for grants to cover permission fees. Gary Ferngren acknowledges the grant of a sabbatical leave for the spring term of 2015, which materially aided in the writing and editing of this volume.

# ESSENTIAL READINGS IN MEDICINE AND RELIGION

# ONE

# The Ancient Near East

## INTRODUCTION

The "ancient Near East" is a phrase that employs a somewhat old-fashioned term to describe the area that includes modern Palestine, Syria, Egypt, Israel, Iran, and Iraq. It has become conventional usage among historians and is still widely used to refer geographically to the Middle East before its conquest by Alexander the Great (356–323 BCE). This chapter includes texts that describe the healing that ancient peoples attributed to divinities in the diverse cultures that constituted the ancient Near East: Mesopotamia from the Sumerian period through the Babylonian, which ended with the Persian conquest of Babylon (c. 3200–539 BCE); Egypt from the union of the Upper and Lower Kingdoms to its conquest by Alexander the Great (c. 3100–332 BCE); and Israel from the exodus out of Egypt (variously dated c. 1450 or c. 1280 BCE) to the Roman destruction of Jerusalem in 70 CE.

Healing in the ancient world took a variety of forms, some secular and some religious or magical. Disease was generally attributed to four kinds of causation. In the first, it was said to be caused by gods or divinities and was often considered to be retributive, that is, inflicted in response to an act that had aroused the displeasure of a god or divine force. In the second type, disease was attributed to demons (minor deities or malevolent spirits). In the third, it was said to be caused by the magic of magicians or sorcerers. Finally, disease was seen to be the result of natural causes that could be observed, for example, in wounds and broken bones. While in some societies one or another model of disease causation was dominant, in most ancient cultures all four were seen as potential causes, and a proper diagnosis was necessary to determine which type was the cause and what kind of treatment would be effective in each instance. In the case of a divinely caused illness, a religious form of healing—such as prayer, sacrifice, or purification—was employed. Exorcism was the usual means of expelling disease-causing demons, though religious healing might also be sought. Magical means—such as amulets or incantations—were used when magic was suspected. Illness caused by natural forces would be treated by natural or medical means, though on occasion by religious healing. In virtually all ancient cultures, these different etiologies, or investigations of the cause of disease, coexisted and complemented one another, sometimes in learned medicine and often in popular or folk medicine.

## Mesopotamia

Mesopotamian or Babylonian religion was polytheistic and based on the worship of personified natural forces. Disease was thought to be caused by intrusive demons, who had to be identified and expelled by incantations [1.4] or purgatives (such as laxatives) [1.2], which were often used together. In the Akkadian period (beginning c. 2350 BCE) gods were called upon against disease-causing demons [1.3], while illness was viewed as divine retribution for sins committed [1.2]. Therapy included confession, in which the sufferer sought to identify the offenses, whether moral or ritual failings, that had brought about the affliction [1.3]. Divination was sometimes used in prognosis (the attempt to forecast the course of an illness) together with the signs and symptoms of various physical afflictions [1.1]. Incantations to Gula, the Babylonian goddess of healing, who was also a physician [1.6], or to a guardian spirit accompanied the medicinal remedies that were administered.

There were two kinds of healers during much of Mesopotamian history, and their professions were complementary. The *mašmaššu* or *āšipu* (the terms were perhaps synonymous), a ritual expert (priest, exorcist, or magician), made the diagnosis and prognosis, while the natural healer, the *asû*, offered drugs and used additional natural and empirical methods, such as cathartics and suppositories. Whether the herbs and minerals used by the asû helped in the patient's recovery is difficult to assess, but what we would today call the "placebo effect" of the āšipu's incantations or amulets may well have helped in the healing.

# Egypt

We know a good deal about Egyptian medicine from a dozen medical texts that have been preserved on papyri. One of the most important, the Edwin Smith Papyrus, dating from about 1600 BCE but with a fragmentary text that was probably compiled two or three hundred years earlier, describes forty-eight cases of injuries to the head, neck, chest, or shoulder (the remainder of the text, which described the other parts of the body, is missing), for which it recommends natural treatments and eight magical incantations. Another is the Papyrus Ebers, which contains the most complete Egyptian collection of treatment recipes and accompanying incantations [1.9]. Incantations were widely used by Egyptian healers, often together with amulets, which they believed could overcome evil forces.

Religion was an essential component of all facets of Egyptian life and culture, including healing. Each part of the body was associated with a god, and a myth assigned the creation of each part of the human body and all animal life to the great god Khnum, who formed them on a pottery wheel [1.8]. Like the Mesopotamians, Egyptians believed that sin could bring about illness, and they sometimes sought the forgiveness of the god they had offended [1.10]. Several gods were associated with healing, including Thoth, the physician of the gods [1.9a]; the goddess Isis [1.9b]; and Imhotep, vizier to Pharaoh Djoser (c. 2650–c. 2575 BCE), who came to be deified as the healing god Ptah and as the god Imouthes. The cult of Imouthes enjoyed popularity until Roman times through incubation, the practice of sleeping overnight in a temple precinct for healing [1.11, 1.12]. Personal cleanliness and hygiene were emphasized in Egyptian medicine as elements of religious purity rather than of sanitation.

Like the Mesopotamians, ancient Egyptians sought the services of several kinds of healers. The *wabw* was a priest of Sekhmet, a goddess of healing, who apparently combined magic and religious healing practices with drug therapy. The *sa.u* was an exorcist or sorcerer who employed recitals and charms, but also drugs, which carried both a magico-religious and an empirical value in Egypt. The third kind of healer was the *swnw*, who was both a priest of the god Thoth and a natural healer. His treatments combined recitals and prayers with drug therapy [1.9a]. The mingling of natural therapy with magical and religious approaches was a characteristic feature of Egyptian medicine. Sometimes a single person combined all three professions.

# Israel

Though the Hebrews (known as Israelites or Jews at different times in their history) shared many of the cultural characteristics of the broader ancient Near Eastern culture, they were distinguished by their religious outlook, which was normatively but not consistently monotheistic. They worshiped Yahweh who, they believed, had entered into a covenant relationship with Israel. His favor to his people was shown by the Torah, which reflected his holy character, revealed his law, and described the worship and moral conduct of both the nation and individual Hebrews. One quality that was to characterize Israel was compassion, or loving kindness, which should be shown to those who were suffering or in need.

The Hebrews believed that disease was sometimes (though not commonly) a consequence of sin, sent by Yahweh. In ancient societies gods dealt with peoples collectively, often punishing a city for the sins of even one person. This is a theme reflected often in the Hebrew Bible. The Israelites, like the early Romans, seem to have had no native tradition of medical healing, perhaps a result of their nomadic background. They sometimes employed physicians from Egypt, although the Egyptians' magic and ritual healing might have been implicitly prohibited by the Torah. The Israelites also used the folk medicine practices that were common in every ancient society (e.g., balm [1.14]), and on occasion they relied on prayer, repentance for wrongdoing, and fasting to seek Yahweh's favor in healing. Although the prominence accorded these religious methods of divine healing in the Hebrew Bible may suggest that they were frequent practices, they were probably regarded as occasional instances of Yahweh's direct intervention. The Hebrews ascribed all healing to Yahweh (Exodus 15:26) and acknowledged that physicians, folk practitioners, and other healers owed their efficacy to him.

The Israelites did not regard demons as the cause of disease until the Second Temple period, when Jews returning from the Babylonian captivity beginning in 538 BCE brought with them a demonic etiology of disease borrowed from the Babylonians. This became a minority view among the Jews, both among the general population and among sectarian groups, such as the Essenes. Most Hebrews held a naturalistic view of disease and illness, even while attributing them theologically at times to Yahweh's chastisement of his people. But their knowledge of disease and medicine remained rudimentary until the introduction of Greek medicine in the Hellenistic period (323–30 BCE). Greek medicine, with its theoretical approach to disease, emphasis on natural causality, use of rational and empirical methods of healing, and view of physicians as professionally trained healers, came over time to be widely accepted. This positive view of medicine can be seen in the well-known praise of physicians in the apocryphal Wisdom of Jesus ben Sira (Ecclesiasticus) (early second century BCE) [1.15].

Like the Mesopotamians, the Hebrews struggled with accounting for suffering, particularly the suffering of the innocent. The book of Job grew out of reflection on this theme and now constitutes the best-known theodicy or divine justification for suffering of the Western world [1.16]. And, like the Egyptians, the Hebrews placed ritual purity high on the list of religious observances and were subject to a detailed series of laws that prohibited unclean or impure animal foods [1.13a]. The so-called Holiness Code also contains extensive regulations for separating from the community those who had contracted leprosy [1.13b], together with detailed provisions for the purification of the people who no longer had the disease, their clothes, and their homes, and the healed people's reentry to the community.

## TEXTS

## Mesopotamia

### 1.1
### A diagnostic and prognostic handbook
JoAnn Scurlock, *Sourcebook for Ancient Mesopotamian Medicine*[1]

*In the eleventh century BCE, a physician named Esagil-kinapli compiled a diagnostic and prognostic handbook that listed the symptoms complained of by patients together with an appropriate diagnosis for each. It consisted of forty clay tablets that were divided into six parts. The first section was devoted to divination. A flexible system was created for diagnosing disease in which physical symptoms were taken into account along with supernatural causes, such as the attack of a demon, god, ghost, or sorcerer. The list begins at the top of the head and proceeds to the feet.*

1. When you approach the patient, [do not approach] the patient until you have cast a spell [over yourself].

2. If you pour water on the patient's face and he does not shudder [and] he does not recognize [one known to him], "hand" of [ . . . ]; he will not get well.

. . .

22–23. If from the middle of his skull it hurts him intensely and his eyelid, his forehead, his eye, his cheek, his neck, his breast, his ⌜nipples⌝? [ . . . ], his legs (and) his ankles all together hurt him continually and (the pain) does not let up despite (lit.: in the face of) the *ăšipu*('s efforts), a ghost afflicts him and [continually] pursues [him].

. . .

41–42. If his head continually afflicts him, his neck continually hurts him intensely, his breast continually hurts him, he continually has a crushing sensation in his chest, [he is continually] and incessantly [troubled], he eats and drinks (but) does not eat and drink again, Ishtar continually pursues him because of a house with four (entrances?) (var. crossroads). For a woman, it is because of well and cup; for the queen or an adolescent girl, it is because of place of mourning and tavern.

43. If his head continually afflicts him and fever continually falls upon him, "hand" of Ishtar.

. . .

45–46. If his head continually afflicts him and fever (has) its seat equally all over (and) when his illness leaves him, he has dizziness and trembles (and) if, when his confusional state comes over him, his mentation is altered so that he wanders about without knowing (where he is) as in affliction by a ghost, Lamashtu afflicts [him]. [He] will come through.

. . .

48–49. If his head trembles, his neck and his spine are bent, he cannot raise his mouth to the words, his saliva continually flows from his mouth, his hands, his legs and his feet all tremble together, (and) when he walks, he falls forward, if [ . . . ] he will not get well.

. . .

57–58. If his head (has) a very hot temperature (and) over the course of a day it leaves him and then (later) it overpowers him (and) flows over him for two days (as in) affliction by a ghost and [his] feet [are cold], (and) when (the fever) releases him, his hands and feet are hot and a cold sweat continually falls on him as in affliction by a ghost, *aḫḫāzu*. If it is prolonged, [he will die].

. . .

61–63. If his head is hot (and) the blood vessel(s) of his temples, his hands and his feet all (seem to) pulsate together, his feet are cold as far as the legs, the bulb of his nose is dark, the undersides of his fingers are unevenly colored with yellow, there are dots of yellow and white in his eyes, both upper and lower eyelids are seized [ . . . ] his breath is seized in his nose so that he makes his breath go out through his mouth, it will make death mount to his throat.

## 1.2
## Purification ritual for a personal-god anxiety
JoAnn Scurlock, *Sourcebook for Ancient Mesopotamian Medicine*[2]

*In seeking treatment for physical illness, the sufferer employed both a religious and a medical approach. If one incurred the anger of a god, it was necessary to undergo a ritual that included purification, which this tablet prescribes. The ritual includes a change of clothes, the burning of incense, libations of water, personal prayer, and (with the appropriate gestures of humility) confession of the wrongdoing that has called forth a god's anger. In this case the person experienced signs of personal anxiety, depression, and stress but without other physical symptoms that would denote an identifiable illness.*

84–97. If a person ponders untruths with his heart, he repeats his words, he is now sleeping, now awake, and he cannot make up his mind (to do anything), the anger of his god is upon him. On a favorable day, that person should purify and wash himself. He should put on a new garment. He should set up one incense burner (burning) *burāšu*-juniper before his god (and) one (burning) *erēnu*-cedar before the god of his city. He should pour out a libation of water. He should kneel. He should pray, and you have him say as follows: "I have altered the brightness [of the moon god]; may your angry heart calm down. May the water that brings relaxation beseech you." He says (this) three times and prostrates himself. If he repeats this [seven?] times, the wrath of his god should be dispelled from him.

## 1.3
## A penitential prayer
JoAnn Scurlock, *Sourcebook for Ancient Mesopotamian Medicine*[3]

*Prayers of confession were an integral part of Mesopotamian medicine because diseases were often attributed not to physiological but to spiritual forces, which sent them as punishment for an offense, either moral or ritual. Illness of any kind was regarded as an evil demon that had seized the sick person, who became the demon's captive. The šigū prayer was a penitential prayer recited aloud and accompanied by the appropriate physical signs of humility and reverence, such as kneeling. Since it was often not possible to discern which god had sent the physical affliction as punishment or from which trespass it had resulted, the confession was general and made to whatever god the penitent had offended and for whichever sin he or she had committed or taboo he or she had transgressed.*

(rev. 7′–20′) If a person wishes to cry a *šigū*-prayer to his god, on a propitious day in the [morning] (and) in the evening, he scatters a sprinkled scatter-offering. This is a scatter-offering. He does not [perform] a ritual hand washing (with it). That person kneels behind the offering arrangement and then [he puts] his arm(s) behind his (back) [and then] he says as follows: "This is the misdeed and sin [which I have committed]. I was negligent; I sinned against my god; I belittled my goddess. I have crossed your boundary, [eaten] what is sacred/offensive to you, trod on what is abomination to you. Whatever I have done, I know very well (that I have done something wrong). My god, release (it); my goddess, remove (it). Make my sins into good deeds." [If] he says this seven times and then kneels, his sin should be dispelled and [he should be able to achieve] whatever he wants.

## 1.4
### A recital against Lamashtu
JoAnn Scurlock, *Sourcebook for Ancient Mesopotamian Medicine*[4]

*Recitals were an integral part of Mesopotamian therapy, according to which disease was attributed not to physiological but to spiritual forces. Illness of any kind could be ascribed to an evil demon that had seized the sick person. This text addresses the Elamite demon Lamashtu, who caused miscarriages through a form of fever, perhaps typhoid. The recital involved the ritual tying of a figurine of Lamashtu to a black dog; this symbolized her marriage so that, with a husband, she would leave the sufferer alone.*

i.11–20. Recitation: Lamashtu, daughter of Anu, by whom the gods swear, Inanna, trustworthy lady, lady of the black-headed people—may you be made to swear by heaven; may you be made to swear by earth. I have married you to a black dog, your slave; I have poured out for you well water (as a libation). Let up! Go away! Withdraw and distance yourself from the body of the infant, son of his god! I have made you swear by Anu and Antu. Ditto (I have made you swear) by Enlil and Ninlil. Ditto (I have made you swear) by Marduk and Anunītum (variant: Sarpanitum). Ditto (I have made you swear) by the great gods of heaven and earth. If you ever return [to] this house (may you be punished)! Spell and Recitation.

. . .

i.22–30. Its ritual: You make a Lamashtu represented as imprisoned. You arrange offerings; you put twelve breads made from unsifted flour before her. You pour out well water for her (as a libation). You marry her to a black dog. For three days you have her sit at the head of the patient. You put the heart of a piglet in [her] mouth. You pour out hot broth for her. You give [her] a wooden *šikkatu*-vessel full of oil. You provide her with [provisions]. You put out dried bread for her. You recite the spell (every day) in the morning, noon, and evening. On the third day you take her out and bury [her] in the corner of a wall.

## 1.5
### A transfer ritual to avert miscarriage
JoAnn Scurlock, *Sourcebook for Ancient Mesopotamian Medicine*[5]

*This recitation, one of three rituals for women who suffered from frequent miscarriages, called for a rite of transfer, in which the woman sought to transmit her inability to carry a child to full term to a pregnant ewe sacred to the gods Šakkan and Dumuzi and to receive in return the ewe's ability to bear offspring.*

(rev. 12′–13′). Ritual for making bring to term a woman who does not bring (her children) to term. You set out a censer (burning) juniper before Gula (Ninkarrak, goddess of healing). You pour out a libation of *miḫḫu*-beer and she (the patient) says as follows.

(rev. 14′–17′). "Ninkarrak, exalted mistress, your merciful mother, may the pregnant ewe of Šakkan and Dumuzi (gods of domestic animals) receive my pregnancy from me and give me her pregnancy. May she receive from me (my) inability to give birth right away and give me her ability to give birth right away."

## 1.6
## Gula, goddess of healing
### *a. Hymn of Gula*
Barbara Bock, *The Healing Goddess Gula*[6]

*This hymn of Gula, the Babylonian goddess of healing, dates from the late second or early first millennium BCE. Gula, also called Ninkarrak [1.6b], is usually depicted surrounded by stars with her dog by her side. The hymn, written from Gula's perspective, begins by praising her exalted status in the universe and the underworld before turning to her celebrated roles in healing and agriculture. It also praises her consort Ninurta in parallel stanzas. The following excerpt is the portion of her two-hundred-line hymn that deals with her role as divine physician. In these few lines, as Barbara Bock writes, "the healing goddess embodies the sum of [Mesopotamian] medical literature."[7]*

> I am the physician, I know how to heal.
> I take along all healing plants, I expel disease.
> I am girded with a bag containing life-giving incantations.
> I carry a scalpel for curing.
> I am giving medication to people:
> The pure bandage soothes the skin sore,
> The soft poultice eases the sickness.
> My very glance at the moribund revives him,
> My mere words make the weak stand up.
> . . .
> I am merciful; even from afar I am listening,
> I bring back the moribund from the netherworld.
> I am girded with a leather bag . . . a scalpel and a knife.
> I am watching over the enfeebled, I examine the sick, I open the skin
>     sore.
> I am the Lady of Life:
> I am the physician, I am the seeress, and I am the exorcist.

## b. Gula appears in a dream to Nabonidus

James B. Pritchard, *Ancient Near Eastern Texts Relating*
*to the Old Testament*[8]

*Nabonidus (556–539 BCE) was the last of the neo-Babylonian kings before Babylon fell to the Persian king Cyrus in 539 BCE. Nabonidus's mother origi-nally came from Haran before moving with her family to Babylon. Nabonidus attained the throne by means of a conspiracy. Called the "royal archaeologist," he was an antiquarian who sought to restore historic temples throughout Mes-opotamia, especially the temple of Sin at Haran. He spent the last years of his reign in Arabia, where he established a new capital at Tema, some 500 miles (805 kilometers) south of Babylon, leaving his son Belshazzar in Babylon to rule in his place. The following text is autobiographical and describes in Nabonidus's own words the appearance of Gula to him in a night vision and her pleading on his behalf for a long life and success against his enemies before the great Babylonian god Marduk, who had not previously been favorably disposed to him.*

### vii

(2–3 lines missing) [*altars* of the planet] Venus, the planet Saturn, the Sing-ing Star . . . the great stars dwelling in heaven, the great witnesses (*of my dream*) I set up for them and prayed to them for a life lasting through many days, permanence of (my) throne, endurance of (my) rule, and that my words might be received favorably before Marduk my lord. (Then) I lay down and beheld in a night(ly vision) the goddess Gula who restores the health of the dead(ly sick) and bestows long life. I prayed to her for lasting life for myself and that she might turn her face towards me. And she actually did turn and looked steadily upon me with her shining face (thus) indicating (her) mercy. I entered the temple . . . into the presence of Nebo, he who extends (the length of) my rule; he placed into my hands the correct scepter, the lawful staff, which (alone) ensures the aggrandizement of the country. I beheld the throne of the goddess Tashmetum (who is) Gula (in the role of) bestower of life. She did present my cause favorably before Marduk, my lord, with re-gard to the lengthening of (my) life into future days and the overthrowing of all opposition. And the wrath of Marduk, my lord, did (eventually) calm down and—full of awe—I dared to praise him; (then) with fervent prayers I approached his sanctuary and (eventually) addressed my prayers to him (directly), telling him my very thoughts as follows: "If I am in reality a king who pleases your heart—and I am not certain (yet), I (still) do not know (this)—one in whose (text: my) hands you, lord of lords, intend to entrust a kingship which is more (important) than that of the kings whom you have nominated in former times to exercise the rule—do make my days last long; (if) I live through long years (lit: if my years grow old), I shall care for the sanctuaries."

## 1.7
### "I will praise the Lord of wisdom"
James B. Pritchard, *Ancient Near Eastern Texts Relating to the Old Testament*[9]

*Several Mesopotamian narratives take the form of theodicies, which address the question of why the just suffer. The best known is called* Ludlul bel néméqi, *after the initial Akkadian words, "I will praise the Lord of wisdom" (that is, Marduk). It is a Mesopotamian analogue to the book of Job and consists of four tablets. The first is very fragmentary. It describes the reversal of fortune of the writer, who was a lord but became a virtual slave with a life marked by much distress. In tablet II he relates how demons have turned his personal gods against him. He has received no help from gods, exorcists, or diviners, and so he examines himself by listing the sins of which he may be guilty. Because every sick person was regarded as a sinner, failure to identify the demon necessitated the discovery of the sin. He searches but cannot find the sins that have brought the punishment of the gods and, like Job, he proclaims in lines 23ff. that he is morally upright. In lines 33ff. he complains that the ways of the gods are beyond finding out. Their values are different from those of humans, and they do not reveal their standards. In tablet II (reverse) the writer gives a moving description of his physical condition brought about by the punishment of the gods. He describes how he suffers the pains of a wretched man, not merely a physical illness but with a deep suffering of the soul that brings with it sleeplessness, indigestion, melancholy, and mourning. Tablet II concludes with his death (lines 46ff.), and tablets III and IV, in which the tone and language differ from the earlier tablets, are likely later additions. In tablet III (reverse) Marduk revokes the curse that brought about the patient's suffering. In tablet IV the writer describes his return to Babylon and the various healing gates through which he enters. He offers gifts, sacrifices, and libations to Marduk and his consort Sarpanit, which gladden their hearts. The moral of the poem, which is*

*slightly abbreviated here, is that the ways of the gods are inexplicable but,*
*although one despairs, in the end the gods will bring deliverance.*

I

I have become like a deaf man. . . .
Once I behaved like a lord, now I have become a slave.
. . .
The fury of my companions destroys me.
. . .
The day is sighing, the night is weeping;
The month is silence, mourning is the year.

II

I have arrived, I have passed beyond life's span.                    (1)
I look about me: evil upon evil!
My affliction increases, right I cannot find.
I implored the god [his personal god], but he did not turn his
    countenance;
I prayed to my goddess, but she did not raise her head.
The diviner through divination did not discern the situation.
Through incense-offering the dream-interpreter did not explain my
    right.
I turned to the necromancer, but he did not enlighten me.
The conjurer through magic did not dispel the wrath against me.
Whence come the evil things everywhere?                              (10)
I looked backwards: persecution, woe!
Like one who did not offer a libation to a god,
And at meal-time did not invoke a goddess,
Who did not bow his face and did not reverence,
In whose mouth prayer and supplication ceased,
For whom the holiday had been eliminated, the *essesu* festival
    [celebrated 4th, 8th, 17th day of the month] has been curtailed,
Who became negligent, despised their images,
Who did not teach his people religion and reverence.
Who did not remember his god, although eating his food,
Who forsook his goddess and did not offer her a libation;            (20)
Nay, worse than one who became proud and forgot his (divine) lord,

Who swore frivolously in the name of his honorable deity—like such
    a one have I become!
Yet I myself was thinking only of prayer and supplication:
Supplication was my concern, sacrifice my rule;
The day of the worship of the gods was my delight,
The day of my goddess' procession was my profit and wealth.
Veneration of the king was my joy,
And I enjoyed music in his honor.
I taught my land to observe the divine ordinances,
To honor the name of the goddess I instructed my people.    (30)
The king's majesty I equated to that of a god,
And reverence for the (royal) palace I inculcated in the troops.
Oh that I only knew that these are well pleasing to a god!
What is good in one's sight is evil for a god.
What is bad in one's mind is good for his god.
Who can understand the counsel of the gods in the midst of heaven?
The plan of a god is deep waters, who can comprehend it?
Where has befuddled mankind ever learned what a god's conduct is?
He who was living yesterday has died today:
Instantly he is made gloomy, suddenly he is crushed.    (40)
One moment he sings a happy song,
And in an instant he will moan like a mourner.
Like day and night their mood changes.
When they are hungry they resemble corpses,
When they are sated they rival their god;
In good luck they speak of ascending to heaven,
When they are afflicted they grumble about going down to the
    underworld.

*II reverse*
The tall [body] they destroy like a wall,    (3)
My broad figure they brought low like a reed.
Like a *sungirtu* (water plant) I was torn away and cast upon my belly.
The *alû* (disease demon) has clothed himself with my body as with a
    garment.
Like a net, sleep has covered me.
My eyes stare without seeing.
My ears are open without hearing.

Faintness has seized my whole body. (10)
A stroke has fallen upon my flesh.
Weakness has taken hold of my hand.
Weariness has fallen upon my knees.

. . .

Death [pursued me] and covered my whole body.
If someone asking for me calls me, I do not answer.
My people weep, I myself no longer exist.
In my mouth a gag is placed,
I hold back the word of my lips. (20)

. . .

Wheat, even though putrid, I eat.
Beer—life divine!—I have eliminated from me.
Extremely long has lasted the distress.
Through starving my appearance . . .
My flesh is flaccid, my blood is [going].
My bones are smashed. . . .
My muscles are inflamed. . . .
I took the bed to the jail, they have blocked (my) exit. (30)
My prison—that is what my house has become.

. . .

I spend the night in my dung, like an ox. (41)
I was soaked like a sheep in my excrements.
My arthritis baffled the conjurer,
And my omens confused the diviner.
The enchanter has not determined the condition of my illness,
And the time (of the end) of my malady the diviner did not give (me).
No god helped, (none) seized my hand;
My goddess showed no mercy, she did not come to my side.
While the grave was still open they took possession of my jewels.
Before I was dead the weeping (for me) was ended. (50)
All my land said, "How sad!"
My ill-wisher heard it, and his countenance shone (with joy);
They brought the good news to the woman who was my ill-wisher, and
    her spirit was delighted.
But I know the day on which my tears will cease,
On which in the midst of the protecting deities their divinity will show
    mercy.

*III reverse*

Out of trouble, through deliverance, I came.                    (66)

The waters of Esagila [the temple of Marduk in Babylon] though weary,
    I set forth in my hands.

Into the mouth of the lion who was devouring me Marduk placed a bit.

Marduk removed the incantation of the one hounding me, turned back
    his lumps.


*IV*

With lowly countenance I entered Esagila [with its twelve gates into
    Babylon]:                                                  (20)

I, who had gone down into the grave, returned to Babylon.

. . .

In the "Welfare Gate" I appeared before Marduk.

In the "Gate of Full Opulence" I kissed the foot of the goddess Sarpanit.

In supplication and imploration I persisted before them.

Sweet-smelling incense smoke I offered to them.

I presented (to them my) produce, gifts, *angub-te*-offerings.

I slew fat oxen, I sacrificed lambs.

I offered a libation of sweet date wine, . . . wine.

I . . . the divine Shedu, to the divine protectors of the walls of Esagila;

With libations I made happy their mood,                        (40)

[With] abundant . . . gladdened their heart.


# Egypt

## 1.8

### Great hymn to Khnum, creator of bodies

Miriam Lichtheim, *Ancient Egyptian Literature*[10]


*Khnum, who was associated with Amon, Re, and Horus, was one of the great-
est gods of Egypt. He was represented in a man's form with a ram's head with
double horns. He was a creator god who continually formed humans and all
living things on a potter's wheel. This reading is a portion of the great hymn to
Khnum from the temple of Esna in Elephantine. The hymn is divided into three
parts. In the first, from which the following is taken, the god is depicted as en-
dowing the human body with all its functions and parts.*

Another hymn to Khnum-Re,
God of the potter's wheel,
Who settled the land by his handiwork;
Who joins in secret,
Who builds soundly,
Who nourishes the nestlings by the breath of his mouth;
Who drenches this land with Nun,
While round sea and great ocean surround him.

He has fashioned gods and men,
He has formed flocks and herds;
He made birds as well as fishes,
He created bulls, engendered cows.
He knotted the flow of blood to the bones,
Formed in his [workshop] as his handiwork,
So the breath of life is within everything,
[Blood bound with semen] in the bones,
To knit the bones from the start.

He makes women give birth when the womb is ready,
So as to open - - - as he wishes;
He soothes suffering by his will,
Relieves throats, lets everyone breathe,
To give life to the young in the womb.

He made hair sprout and tresses grow,
Fastened the skin over the limbs;
He built the skull, formed the cheeks,
To furnish shape to the image [i.e., the human figure].
He opened the eyes, hollowed the ears,
He made the body inhale air;
He formed the mouth for eating,
Made the gorge [i.e., throat] for swallowing.

He also formed the tongue to speak,
The jaws to open, the gullet to drink,
The throat to swallow and spit.

The spine to give support,
The testicles to [move],
The [arm] to act with vigor,
The rear [the anal area] to perform its task.
The gullet to devour,
Hands and fingers to do their work,
The heart to lead.
The loins to support the phallus
In the act of begetting.
The frontal organs to consume things,
The rear to aerate the entrails [i.e., at defecation],
Likewise to sit at ease,
And sustain the entrails [i.e., prevent defecation] at night.
The male member to beget,
The womb to conceive,
And increase generations in Egypt.
The bladder to make water,
The virile member to eject
When it swells between the thighs.
The shins to step,
The legs to tread,
The bones doing their task,
By the will of his heart.

## 1.9
### Recitals before medical treatment
Bendix Ebbell, *The Papyrus Ebers*[11]

*The Papyrus Ebers is the most complete of the several papyri with medical information that have come down to us. Although this compilation of treatments probably dates from c. 1550 BCE, much of the information that it preserves is older, perhaps as early as the Old Kingdom. It contains some seven hundred recipes not generally found in Babylonian texts. Each is accompanied by an incantation. The recommendations incorporate the three methods of treatment commonly found in Egyptian medicine: drugs, operations, and magical spells. The text begins with three recitals to use before medical treatment.*

## a. Recital upon treating limbs

The beginning of a recital on applying a remedy to any limb of a man: I have come from Heliopolis with the old ones in the temple, the possessors of protection, the rulers of eternity; assuredly, I have come from Sais with the mother of the gods. They have given me their protection. I have formulae composed by the lord of the universe in order to expel afflictions (caused) by a god or goddess, by dead man or woman etc., which are in this my head, in this my nape, in these my shoulders, in this my flesh, in these my limbs, and in order to punish the accuser, the head of them who cause decay to enter into this my flesh and feebleness (?) into these my limbs as something entering into this my flesh, in this my head, in these my shoulders, in (this) my body, in these my limbs. I belong to Rê; he has said: "I will save him from his enemies, and Thoth shall be his guide, he who lets writing speak and has composed the books; he gives to the skillful, to the physicians who accompany him, skill to cure. The one whom the god loves, him he shall keep alive." It is I whom the god loves, and he shall keep me alive.

—Spoken when applying remedies to any limb of a man which is ill. Really excellent, (proved) many times!

## b. Recital upon loosening a bandage

Another recital for loosening any bandage: Loosened was the loosened one by Isis, Horus was loosened by Isis from the evils done to him by his brother Seth, when he killed his father Osiris. Oh Isis, great in sorcery! Mayst thou loosen me, mayst thou deliver me from everything bad and evil and vicious, from afflictions (caused) by a god or goddess, from dead man or woman, from male or female adversary who will oppose me, like thy loosening and thy delivering with thy son Horus. For I have entered into the fire and have come forth from the water, I will not fall into this day's trap. I have spoken (and now) I am young and am [ . . . ].—Oh Rê, speak over thine (Uraeus) serpent! Osiris, call over what came out of thee! Rê speaks over his (Uraeus) serpent, Osiris calls over what came out of him. Lo, thou hast saved me from everything bad and evil and vicious, from afflictions (caused) by a god or goddess, from dead man or woman etc.

—Really excellent, (proved) many times!

### c. Recital upon administering a drug

Recital on drinking a remedy: Come remedy! Come thou who expellest (evil) things in this my stomach and in these my limbs! The spell is powerful over the remedy. Repeat it backwards! Dost thou remember that Horus and Seth have been conducted to the big palace at Heliopolis, when there was negotiated of Seth's testicles with Horus, and he shall get well like one who is on earth. He does all that he may wish like these gods who are there.

—Spoken when drinking a remedy. Really excellent, (proved) many times!

### 1.10
### A blind man seeks healing from Ptah
T. Eric Peet, *A Comparative Study of the Literatures of Egypt, Palestine, and Mesopotamia*[12]

*Egyptians believed that disease often reflected the breakdown of harmony between the sick person and some aspect of the world of spirits or the gods. Perhaps he or she had experienced some evil magic or the anger of some divinity. There was in Egyptian religion a strong moral element, as seen most clearly in the Negative Confession of the Book of the Dead. Sinning resulted in the gods turning against one. In the following prayer, a man was guilty of the sin of swearing falsely by Ptah, the god of truth, and as a consequence he was struck with blindness. He confesses his sin, displays penitence, and asks the god for healing.*

I am a man who swore falsely by Ptah, Lord of Truth;

And he caused me to behold darkness by day.
I will declare his might to him that knows him not and to him that
  knows him,
To small and great.
Be ye ware of Ptah, Lord of Truth.
Lo, he will not overlook the deed of any man.
Refrain ye from uttering the name of Ptah falsely;
Lo, he that uttereth it falsely,
Lo, he falleth.
He caused me to be as the dogs of the street,
I being in his hand:

He caused men and gods to mark me,
I being as a man that has wrought abomination against his Lord.
Righteous was Ptah, Lord of Truth, toward me,
When he chastised me.
Be merciful to me; look upon me, that thou mayest be merciful.

## 1.11
## Healing in the shrine of Imouthes
### J. Worth Estes, *The Medical Skills of Ancient Egypt*[13]

*The semilegendary Imhotep was the vizier, or chief minister, of Pharaoh Djoser.*
*He was credited with many achievements, including being a physician. An*
*architect, he designed the first pyramid in Egypt, the step pyramid at Saqqara.*
*A religious cult grew up around his memory, and he became assimilated with*
*the Greek healing god Asklepios and called Imouthes. The following abbrevi-*
*ated text dates from the second century CE; he was still worshiped in Egypt*
*during Roman times, three thousand years after his death, and healing and*
*fertility were still sought from his shrine.*

I was pregnant by him [my husband] three times but did not bear a male
child, only three daughters. I prayed together with the high priest to the
majesty of the god of great wonders, effective in deeds, who gives a son to
him who has none: Imhotep Son of Ptah.

He heard our pleas, he harkened to his prayers. The majesty of this god
came to the head of the high priest in a revelation. He said: "Let a great
work be done in the holy of holies of Ankhtawi, the place where my body is
hidden. As reward for it I shall give you a male child."

When he [my husband] awakened from this he kissed the ground to the
august god. . . . He performed the opening of the mouth for the august god.
He made a great sacrifice of all good things. . . . In return [the god] made me
conceive a male child.

He was born . . . on the Offering-feast of the august god Imhotep Son of
Ptah. [The child's] appearance was like that of [Imhotep]. There was jubilation
over him by the people of Memphis. He was given the name of Imhotep. . . .
Everyone rejoiced over him.

## 1.12
## Incubation in the temple of Imouthes
J. Worth Estes, *The Medical Skills of Ancient Egypt*[14]

*The following excerpt, which also dates from the second century CE, relates a case of healing by incubation, which was practiced in Egypt centuries before it became common in healing temples in Greece and elsewhere. This Greek text, part of an extensive library discovered on the west bank of the Nile near the site of the village of Oxyrhynchus, demonstrates the continuing practice of incubation in Egypt during Roman times.*

It was night, when every living creature was asleep except those in pain, but divinity showed itself the more effectively; a violent fever burned me, and I was convulsed with loss of breath and coughing, owing to the pain proceeding from my side. Heavy in the head with my troubles I was lapsing half-conscious into sleep [at a temple, probably that of Imhotep at Memphis], and my mother, as a mother would for her child [although the patient had earlier described himself as aged], . . . was sitting without enjoying even a short period of slumber, when suddenly she perceived—it was no dream or sleep, for her eyes were open immovably, though not seeing clearly, for a divine and terrifying vision came to her, easily preventing her from observing the god himself or his servants, whichever it was. In any case there was someone whose height was more than human, clothed in shining raiment and carrying in his left hand a book, who after merely regarding me two or three times from head to foot disappeared. When she had recovered herself, she tried, still trembling, to wake me, and finding the fever had left me and that much sweat was pouring off me, did reverence to the manifestation of the god, and then wiped me and made me more collected. . . . everything that she saw in the vision appeared to me in dreams. After these pains in my side had ceased and the god had given me yet another assuaging cure, I proclaimed his benefits. [This was not enough for the god, and he forced the writer to return to an earlier promise to write a book about the god and his cult, because] a written record is an undying [reward] of gratitude, from time to time renewing its youth in the memory. Every Greek tongue will tell thy story, and every Greek man will worship the son of Ptah, Imouthes [i.e., Imhotep/Asklepios].

# Israel

## 1.13
## The Holiness Code

*The Holiness Code consists of chapters 11–16 of the book of Leviticus, the third book of the Torah or Pentateuch, the law of Moses. It prescribes the ways in which defilement could come about in Hebrew life. Though called the Holiness Code, it deals with ritual, not moral, purity. For the Hebrews ritual defilement could occur in four ways: by eating unclean foods, such as pork; by contracting leprosy; by contact with a dead body; and by the discharge of bodily fluids associated with reproduction, such as semen or menstrual flow. The best-known regulations of the code, the dietary laws, circumscribed the eating of "unclean" foods. A traditional interpretation of these regulations is that certain prohibited fish carry harmful parasites, while birds of prey, being carnivorous, carry harmful diseases. According to this view the prohibition against eating unclean animals represents an empirical folk understanding of hygiene. It appears, however, that consuming the fowl, fish, or animals mentioned in the code carries few, if any, health risks. Mary Douglas suggests that the code was intended to define the boundaries of Hebrew sacred space, establishing conduct that produced and maintained a distinct culture separating Israel from the surrounding pagan nations, which might negatively influence its religious and moral culture.[15]*

### a. Clean and unclean animals
Book of Leviticus[16]

11 And the LORD spoke to Moses and Aaron, saying to them, ² Speak to the people of Israel, saying:

From among all the land animals, these are the creatures that you may eat. ³ Any animal that has divided hoofs and is cleft-footed and chews the cud—such you may eat. ⁴ But among those that chew the cud or have divided hoofs, you shall not eat the following: the camel, for even though it chews the cud, it does not have divided hoofs; it is unclean to you. . . . ⁷ The pig, for even though it has divided hoofs and is cleft-footed, it does not chew the cud; it is unclean to you. ⁸ Of their flesh you shall not eat, and their carcasses you shall not touch; they are unclean for you.

⁹ These you may eat, of all that are in the waters. Everything in the waters that has fins and scales, whether in the seas or in the streams—such you may eat. ¹⁰ But anything in the seas or the streams that does not have fins and scales, of the swarming creatures in the waters and among all the other living creatures that are in the waters—they are detestable to you ¹¹ and detestable they shall remain. Of their flesh you shall not eat, and their carcasses you shall regard as detestable. . . .

²⁴ By these you shall become unclean; whoever touches the carcass of any of them shall be unclean until the evening, ²⁵ and whoever carries any part of the carcass of any of them shall wash his clothes and be unclean until the evening. ²⁶ Every animal that has divided hoofs but is not cleft-footed or does not chew the cud is unclean for you; everyone who touches one of them shall be unclean. ²⁷ All that walk on their paws, among the animals that walk on all fours, are unclean for you; whoever touches the carcass of any of them shall be unclean until the evening, ²⁸ and the one who carries the carcass shall wash his clothes and be unclean until the evening; they are unclean for you. . . . ³² And anything upon which any of them falls when they are dead shall be unclean, whether an article of wood or cloth or skin or sacking, any article that is used for any purpose; it shall be dipped into water, and it shall be unclean until the evening, and then it shall be clean. ³³ And if any of them falls into any earthen vessel, all that is in it shall be unclean, and you shall break the vessel. ³⁴ Any food that could be eaten shall be unclean if water from any such vessel comes upon it; and any liquid that could be drunk shall be unclean if it was in any such vessel. ³⁵ Everything on which any part of the carcass falls shall be unclean; whether an oven or stove, it shall be broken in pieces; they are unclean, and shall remain unclean for you. ³⁶ But a spring or a cistern holding water shall be clean, while whatever touches the carcass in it shall be unclean. ³⁷ If any part of their carcass falls upon any seed set aside for sowing, it is clean; ³⁸ but if water is put on the seed and any part of their carcass falls on it, it is unclean for you.

³⁹ If an animal of which you may eat dies, anyone who touches its carcass shall be unclean until the evening. ⁴⁰ Those who eat of its carcass shall wash their clothes and be unclean until the evening; and those who carry the carcass shall wash their clothes and be unclean until the evening.

⁴¹ All creatures that swarm upon the earth are detestable; they shall not be eaten.

⁴² Whatever moves on its belly, and whatever moves on all fours, or whatever has many feet, all the creatures that swarm upon the earth, you shall

not eat; for they are detestable. [43] You shall not make yourselves detestable with any creature that swarms; you shall not defile yourselves with them, and so become unclean. [44] For I am the LORD your God; sanctify yourselves therefore, and be holy, for I am holy.

### b. Laws regarding leprosy
Book of Leviticus[17]

*Biblical leprosy as described in the Pentateuch appears to have encompassed a spectrum of lesions and thus was broader than Hansen's disease (modern leprosy), which affects the skin and peripheral nervous system. The Hebrew word za'arath (Greek, lepra) refers to a scaly condition that could affect not merely the skin, but also clothing and the walls of a house. The vagueness of the symptoms in our sources makes it difficult to differentiate the various conditions that were subsumed under the term, but elephantiasis was among them, and they probably included ringworm and other fungal conditions. Physical disfigurement may or may not fully explain the revulsion that the condition elicited, and the reason for the association of leprosy with ritual defilement (uncleanness) in Hebrew culture is not clear. The quarantining of the affected persons described here was not apparently intended to prevent the spread of the disease as much as to prevent spiritual defilement within the community of Israel.*

13 The LORD spoke to Moses and Aaron, saying: [2] When a person has on the skin of his body a swelling or an eruption or a spot, and it turns into a leprous disease on the skin of his body, he shall be brought to Aaron the priest or to one of his sons the priests. [3] The priest shall examine the disease on the skin of his body, and if the hair in the diseased area has turned white and the disease appears to be deeper than the skin of his body, it is a leprous disease; after the priest has examined him he shall pronounce him ceremonially unclean. [4] But if the spot is white in the skin of his body, and appears no deeper than the skin, and the hair in it has not turned white, the priest shall confine the diseased person for seven days. [5] The priest shall examine him on the seventh day, and if he sees that the disease is checked and the disease has not spread in the skin, then the priest shall confine him seven days more. [6] The priest shall examine him again on the seventh day, and if the disease has abated and the disease has not spread in the skin, the priest shall pronounce him clean; it is only an eruption; and he shall wash his

clothes, and be clean. [7] But if the eruption spreads in the skin after he has shown himself to the priest for his cleansing, he shall appear again before the priest. [8] The priest shall make an examination, and if the eruption has spread in the skin, the priest shall pronounce him unclean; it is a leprous disease. . . .

[45] The person who has the leprous disease shall wear torn clothes and let the hair of his head be disheveled; and he shall cover his upper lip and cry out, "Unclean, unclean." [46] He shall remain unclean as long as he has the disease; he is unclean. He shall live alone; his dwelling shall be outside the camp.

[47] Concerning clothing: when a leprous disease appears in it, in woolen or linen cloth, [48] in warp or woof of linen or wool, or in a skin or in anything made of skin, [49] if the disease shows greenish or reddish in the garment, whether in warp or woof or in skin or in anything made of skin, it is a leprous disease and shall be shown to the priest. [50] The priest shall examine the disease, and put the diseased article aside for seven days. [51] He shall examine the disease on the seventh day. If the disease has spread in the cloth, in warp or woof, or in the skin, whatever be the use of the skin, this is a spreading leprous disease; it is unclean. [52] He shall burn the clothing, whether diseased in warp or woof, woolen or linen, or anything of skin, for it is a spreading leprous disease; it shall be burned in fire.

[53] If the priest makes an examination, and the disease has not spread in the clothing, in warp or woof or in anything of skin, [54] the priest shall command them to wash the article in which the disease appears, and he shall put it aside seven days more. [55] The priest shall examine the diseased article after it has been washed. If the diseased spot has not changed color, though the disease has not spread, it is unclean; you shall burn it in fire, whether the leprous spot is on the inside or on the outside.

[56] If the priest makes an examination, and the disease has abated after it is washed, he shall tear the spot out of the cloth, in warp or woof, or out of skin. [57] If it appears again in the garment, in warp or woof, or in anything of skin, it is spreading; you shall burn with fire that in which the disease appears. [58] But the cloth, warp or woof, or anything of skin from which the disease disappears when you have washed it, shall then be washed a second time, and it shall be clean.

## 1.14
## Jeremiah grieves for his people
Book of Jeremiah[18]

*Jeremiah prophesied during the reigns of the last four kings of Judah, from 626 BCE to the fall of Jerusalem in 586 BCE. In a period of national moral decline, he summoned the people to repent of their sins. Called the "weeping prophet," Jeremiah mourned the lack of genuine repentance on the part of his people and warned them of God's coming judgment. This moving passage describes the prophet's heartbreak in medical terms. He refers to both balm (balsam), a therapeutic substance grown in Gilead, which was perhaps an aromatic spice or gum, and* rapha, *the Hebrew word for healer, metaphorically indicating that neither medicine nor physician can be found to heal the fatal spiritual wound of a people who are facing their last days. They have lost one chance after another for deliverance (symbolized by the passing of the seasons) and now face despair. There is no balm for such wounds, no healing, and indeed none is offered.*

[18] My joy is gone, grief is upon me,
my heart is sick.
[19] Hark, the cry of my poor people
from far and wide in the land:
"Is the LORD not in Zion?
Is her King not in her?"
("Why have they provoked me to anger with their images,
with their foreign idols?")
[20] "The harvest is past, the summer is ended,
and we are not saved."
[21] For the hurt of my poor people I am hurt,
I mourn, and dismay has taken hold of me.
[22] Is there no balm in Gilead?
Is there no physician there?
Why then has the health of my poor people
not been restored?

## 1.15
## The physician as a servant of Yahweh
Book of Ecclesiasticus[19]

*The earliest mention of a Jewish medical profession is found in the Wisdom of Jesus ben Sira (Sirach), traditionally known as Ecclesiasticus, which was composed in Hebrew in Palestine early in the second century BCE and later translated into Greek by the grandson of the author. After the conquest of Palestine by Alexander the Great, Greek culture—including Greek medicine with its new emphasis on physical health and theoretical medicine—entered Hebrew life. Ben Sira urges his readers to honor the physician as a servant of God, who gives him his skill. But while employing medicine for healing, the people should place their dependence on God because it is he who ultimately heals. The physician, too, must look to God for a successful diagnosis and the ability to provide treatment that will save life.*

38 Honor physicians for their services,
for the LORD created them;
² for their gift of healing comes from the Most High,
and they are rewarded by the king.
³ The skill of physicians makes them distinguished,
and in the presence of the great they are admired.
⁴ The LORD created medicines out of the earth,
and the sensible will not despise them.
⁵ Was not water made sweet with a tree
in order that its power might be known?
⁶ And he gave skill to human beings
that he might be glorified in his marvelous works.
⁷ By them the physician heals and takes away pain;
⁸ the pharmacist makes a mixture from them.
God's works will never be finished;
and from him health spreads over all the earth.
⁹ My child, when you are ill, do not delay,
but pray to the LORD, and he will heal you.
¹⁰ Give up your faults and direct your hands rightly,
and cleanse your heart from all sin.
¹¹ Offer a sweet-smelling sacrifice, and a memorial portion of choice flour,
and pour oil on your offering, as much as you can afford.

¹² Then give the physician his place, for the LORD created him;
do not let him leave you, for you need him.
¹³ There may come a time when recovery lies in the hands of physicians,
¹⁴ for they too pray to the LORD
that he grant them success in diagnosis
and in healing, for the sake of preserving life.
¹⁵ He who sins against his Maker,
will be defiant toward the physician.

## 1.16
## The suffering of Job

*The book of Job is the best-known theodicy in Western literature. It deals with the age-old problem of why the righteous suffer. While it has analogies in two Mesopotamian theodicies, the* Ludlul bel nēméqi *("I Will Praise the Lord of Wisdom" [1.7]) and "The Man and His God," it holds a unique place in the religious literature of Western civilization. The anonymous work belongs to the tradition of wisdom literature in the Hebrew Bible, but its chronological and geographical vagueness makes it impossible to date. While its theme of human suffering is addressed by the two Mesopotamian theodicies, the answers they give to the problem reflect the fatalism of the Mesopotamian outlook in which life was governed by the capricious will of the gods. In the case of Job, the answer to the question of justice raised by the undeserved suffering of a man who has committed no sin is given in the last chapter, in which Job acknowledges Yahweh's sovereignty over all life and repents (42:1–6), while also stating that he has drawn closer to Yahweh as a result of his suffering (verse 5).*

### a. Prologue: Job and his family
Book of Job²⁰

*At the beginning Job is described as a prosperous man of sincere piety and great moral virtue who honors God in an early but undated culture.*

1 There was once a man in the land of Uz whose name was Job. That man was blameless and upright, one who feared God and turned away from evil. ² There were born to him seven sons and three daughters. ³ He had seven thousand sheep, three thousand camels, five hundred yoke of oxen, five

hundred donkeys, and very many servants; so that this man was the greatest of all the people of the east. ⁴ His sons used to go and hold feasts in one another's houses in turn; and they would send and invite their three sisters to eat and drink with them. ⁵ And when the feast days had run their course, Job would send and sanctify them, and he would rise early in the morning and offer burnt offerings according to the number of them all; for Job said, "It may be that my children have sinned, and cursed God in their hearts." This is what Job always did.

### b. Satan afflicts Job with boils
Book of Job²¹

*Chapter 2 describes a dramatic scene in heaven in which angels appear before God to give an account of their activities. Among them is Satan. When God presents Job as a blameless and upright man, Satan replies that if Job is struck down with disease (he has already lost his family and material goods) he will curse God. God gives Satan permission to do so, but commands him to spare Job's life. Although Satan afflicts Job with boils, Job refuses to curse God. When his three friends hear of the calamities he has suffered they come to comfort him, first following the Hebrew practice of sitting in silence for seven days in an attitude of mourning.*

2 One day the heavenly beings came to present themselves before the LORD, and Satan also came among them to present himself before the LORD. ² The LORD said to Satan, "Where have you come from?" Satan answered the LORD, "From going to and fro on the earth, and from walking up and down on it." ³ The LORD said to Satan, "Have you considered my servant Job? There is no one like him on the earth, a blameless and upright man who fears God and turns away from evil. He still persists in his integrity, although you incited me against him, to destroy him for no reason." ⁴ Then Satan answered the LORD, "Skin for skin! All that people have they will give to save their lives. ⁵ But stretch out your hand now and touch his bone and his flesh, and he will curse you to your face." ⁶ The LORD said to Satan, "Very well, he is in your power; only spare his life."

⁷ So Satan went out from the presence of the LORD, and inflicted loathsome sores on Job from the sole of his foot to the crown of his head. ⁸ Job took a potsherd with which to scrape himself, and sat among the ashes.

⁹ Then his wife said to him, "Do you still persist in your integrity? Curse God, and die." ¹⁰ But he said to her, "You speak as any foolish woman would speak. Shall we receive the good at the hand of God, and not receive the bad?" In all this Job did not sin with his lips.

¹¹ Now when Job's three friends heard of all these troubles that had come upon him, each of them set out from his home—Eliphaz the Temanite, Bildad the Shuhite, and Zophar the Naamathite. They met together to go and console and comfort him. ¹² When they saw him from a distance, they did not recognize him, and they raised their voices and wept aloud; they tore their robes and threw dust in the air upon their heads. ¹³ They sat with him on the ground seven days and seven nights, and no one spoke a word to him, for they saw that his suffering was very great.

### c. Job curses the day he was born
Book of Job[22]

*While Job refuses to curse Yahweh, he eventually utters a lamentation for the day of his birth. It takes the familiar ancient Near Eastern form of mourning, which comes naturally to a man who has suffered the loss of his family, property, and health. With great poignancy he seeks to understand why all his misfortunes have happened.*

¹¹ "Why did I not die at birth,
come forth from the womb and expire?
¹² Why were there knees to receive me,
or breasts for me to suck?
¹³ Now I would be lying down and quiet;
I would be asleep; then I would be at rest
¹⁴ with kings and counselors of the earth
who rebuild ruins for themselves,
¹⁵ or with princes who have gold,
who fill their houses with silver.
¹⁶ Or why was I not buried like a stillborn child,
like an infant that never sees the light?
¹⁷ There the wicked cease from troubling,
and there the weary are at rest.
¹⁸ There the prisoners are at ease together;
they do not hear the voice of the taskmaster.

¹⁹ The small and the great are there,
and the slaves are free from their masters.
²⁰ Why is light given to one in misery,
and life to the bitter in soul,
²¹ who long for death, but it does not come,
and dig for it more than for hidden treasures;
²² who rejoice exceedingly,
and are glad when they find the grave?
²³ Why is light given to one who cannot see the way,
whom God has fenced in?
²⁴ For my sighing comes like my bread,
and my groanings are poured out like water.
²⁵ Truly the thing that I fear comes upon me,
and what I dread befalls me.
²⁶ I am not at ease, nor am I quiet;
I have no rest; but trouble comes."

### d. Eliphaz speaks: Job has sinned
Book of Job²³

*After holding sympathetic silence out of respect for Job's calamities, Eliphaz speaks to Job. He begins tactfully by praising Job for his encouragement of those who have experienced difficulties, but now that suffering has come on him Job cannot bear it. Eliphaz's words convey the conventional theodicy of the ancient Near East: God helps those who are good and punishes those who are wicked. Yahweh is perfect, and those who have offended his law must expect to suffer. If Job believes that he is innocent, then he must accept the corollary that God is unjust.*

4 Then Eliphaz the Temanite answered:
² "If one ventures a word with you, will you be offended?
But who can keep from speaking?
³ See, you have instructed many;
you have strengthened the weak hands.
⁴ Your words have supported those who were stumbling,
and you have made firm the feeble knees.
⁵ But now it has come to you, and you are impatient;
it touches you, and you are dismayed.

⁶ Is not your fear of God your confidence,
and the integrity of your ways your hope?"

### e. Eliphaz continues: If Job repents, God will deliver him
Book of Job[24]

*Eliphaz continues his monologue by calling on Job to repent. Yahweh's mercy is inexhaustible, and though he humbles the proud he rescues those who are in need. He has struck Job with suffering, but he will deliver him if Job calls upon Yahweh. God responds to those who seek him, and he will send remedies for disasters. There is nothing in Eliphaz's speech that is inconsistent with the theology of the Old Testament, and in another context it would go unchallenged. But it does not comfort Job, who believes that he has done nothing to merit the suffering that Yahweh has brought upon him.*

5 "Call now; is there anyone who will answer you?
To which of the holy ones will you turn?
² Surely vexation kills the fool,
and jealousy slays the simple.
³ I have seen fools taking root,
but suddenly I cursed their dwelling.
⁴ Their children are far from safety,
they are crushed in the gate,
and there is no one to deliver them.
⁵ The hungry eat their harvest,
and they take it even out of the thorns;
and the thirsty pant after their wealth.
⁶ For misery does not come from the earth,
nor does trouble sprout from the ground;
⁷ but human beings are born to trouble
just as sparks fly upward.
⁸ As for me, I would seek God,
and to God I would commit my cause.
⁹ He does great things and unsearchable,
marvelous things without number.
¹⁰ He gives rain on the earth
and sends waters on the fields;

<sup>11</sup> he sets on high those who are lowly,
and those who mourn are lifted to safety.
<sup>12</sup> He frustrates the devices of the crafty,
so that their hands achieve no success.
<sup>13</sup> He takes the wise in their own craftiness;
and the schemes of the wily are brought to a quick end.
<sup>14</sup> They meet with darkness in the daytime,
and grope at noonday as in the night.
<sup>15</sup> But he saves the needy from the sword of their mouth,
from the hand of the mighty.
<sup>16</sup> So the poor have hope,
and injustice shuts its mouth.
<sup>17</sup> How happy is the one whom God reproves;
therefore do not despise the discipline of the Almighty.
<sup>18</sup> For he wounds, but he binds up;
he strikes, but his hands heal.
<sup>19</sup> He will deliver you from six troubles;
in seven no harm shall touch you.
<sup>20</sup> In famine he will redeem you from death,
and in war from the power of the sword.
<sup>21</sup> You shall be hidden from the scourge of the tongue,
and shall not fear destruction when it comes.
<sup>22</sup> At destruction and famine you shall laugh,
and shall not fear the wild animals of the earth.
<sup>23</sup> For you shall be in league with the stones of the field,
and the wild animals shall be at peace with you.
<sup>24</sup> You shall know that your tent is safe,
you shall inspect your fold and miss nothing.
<sup>25</sup> You shall know that your descendants will be many,
and your offspring like the grass of the earth.
<sup>26</sup> You shall come to your grave in ripe old age,
as a shock of grain comes up to the threshing floor in its season.
<sup>27</sup> See, we have searched this out; it is true.
Hear, and know it for yourself."

### f. Job responds: My suffering is without end
Book of Job[25]

*Job replies to Eliphaz, who has offered words that, while true as a general state-ment of Hebrew theodicy, give him no comfort. Job has searched his heart for any trace of moral failing (as did the Mesopotamians who sought explanations for their suffering), and he is convinced that God has no reason to bring retri-bution. He describes the agony of one whose pain and suffering deprive him of any physical comfort, even of sleep (verse 4). His desire is to see and experience Yahweh, who has abandoned him so that he has become a burden to himself (verse 20).*

7 "Do not human beings have a hard service on earth,
and are not their days like the days of a laborer?
[2] Like a slave who longs for the shadow,
and like laborers who look for their wages,
[3] so I am allotted months of emptiness,
and nights of misery are apportioned to me.
[4] When I lie down I say, 'When shall I rise?'
But the night is long,
and I am full of tossing until dawn.
[5] My flesh is clothed with worms and dirt;
my skin hardens, then breaks out again.
[6] My days are swifter than a weaver's shuttle,
and come to their end without hope.
[7] Remember that my life is a breath;
my eye will never again see good.
[8] The eye that beholds me will see me no more;
while your eyes are upon me, I shall be gone.
[9] As the cloud fades and vanishes,
so those who go down to Sheol do not come up;
[10] they return no more to their houses,
nor do their places know them any more.
[11] Therefore I will not restrain my mouth;
I will speak in the anguish of my spirit;
I will complain in the bitterness of my soul.
[12] Am I the Sea, or the Dragon,
that you set a guard over me?

¹³ When I say, 'My bed will comfort me,
my couch will ease my complaint,'
¹⁴ then you scare me with dreams
and terrify me with visions,
¹⁵ so that I would choose strangling
and death rather than this body.
¹⁶ I loathe my life; I would not live forever.
Let me alone, for my days are a breath.
¹⁷ What are human beings, that you make so much of them,
that you set your mind on them,
¹⁸ visit them every morning,
test them every moment?
¹⁹ Will you not look away from me for a while,
let me alone until I swallow my spittle?
²⁰ If I sin, what do I do to you, you watcher of humanity?
Why have you made me your target?
Why have I become a burden to you?
²¹ Why do you not pardon my transgression
and take away my iniquity?
For now I shall lie in the earth;
you will seek me, but I shall not be."

### g. Job is humbled and satisfied
Book of Job²⁶

*Most of the book of Job consists of dialogue between Job and his friends. In the end, God answers Job's complaint out of a whirlwind by asking a series of unanswerable questions (chs. 38–41) that reduce him to silence and demonstrate the power and sovereignty of Yahweh, who acts according to his own will and is not accountable to human beings. Job is overwhelmed, not by his sin, but by questioning the ways of Yahweh. He repents and acknowledges his acceptance of Yahweh's will. His repentance and reconciliation with Yahweh bring about a deeper understanding of God's ways and a renewed fellowship with him (42:5–6). In the end, Job's fortunes are restored twofold, as a gift of God's grace.*

42 Then Job answered the LORD:
² "I know that you can do all things,
and that no purpose of yours can be thwarted.

³ 'Who is this that hides counsel without knowledge?'
Therefore I have uttered what I did not understand,
things too wonderful for me, which I did not know.
⁴ 'Hear, and I will speak;
I will question you, and you declare to me.'
⁵ I had heard of you by the hearing of the ear,
but now my eye sees you;
⁶ therefore I despise myself,
and repent in dust and ashes."

. . .

¹⁰ And the LORD restored the fortunes of Job when he had prayed for his
friends; and the LORD gave Job twice as much as he had before. ¹¹ Then
there came to him all his brothers and sisters and all who had known
him before, and they ate bread with him in his house; they showed him
sympathy and comforted him for all the evil that the LORD had brought
upon him; and each of them gave him a piece of money and
a gold ring. ¹² The LORD blessed the latter days of Job more than his
beginning; and he had fourteen thousand sheep, six thousand camels, a
thousand yoke of oxen, and a thousand donkeys. ¹³ He also had seven
sons and three daughters. ¹⁴ He named the first Jemimah, the second
Keziah, and the third Keren-happuch. ¹⁵ In all the land there were no
women so beautiful as Job's daughters; and their father gave them an
inheritance along with their brothers. ¹⁶ After this Job lived one
hundred and forty years, and saw his children, and his children's
children, four generations. ¹⁷ And Job died, old and full of days.

## NOTES

1. Scurlock, *Sourcebook*, 18–21.
2. Ibid., 661.
3. Ibid., 664.
4. Ibid., 682.
5. Ibid., 690.
6. Bock, *Healing Goddess Gula*, 2–3, lines 79–87, 178–83.
7. Ibid., 3.
8. Pritchard, *Ancient Near Eastern Texts*, 310.
9. Ibid., 434–37.
10. Miriam Lichtheim, *Ancient Egyptian Literature: A Book of Readings*, vol. 3: *The Late Period* (Berkeley: University of California Press, 1980), 112–13. Copyright © 1980, 2006 by the Regents of the University of California.

11. Ebbell, *Papyrus Ebers*, 29–30.

12. Peet, *Comparative Study*, 89.

13. Estes, *Medical Skills of Ancient Egypt*, 131. See also Lichtheim, *Ancient Egyptian Literature*, 62.

14. Estes, *Medical Skills of Ancient Egypt*, 123–24. See also Grenfell and Hunt, *Oxyrhynchus Papyrus*, 221.

15. For more on Mary Douglas, see Gary B. Ferngren, *Medicine and Religion* (Baltimore: Johns Hopkins University Press, 2014).

16. Leviticus 11:1–4, 7–11, 24–28, 32–44.

17. Leviticus 13:1–8, 45–58.

18. Jeremiah 8:18–22.

19. Sirach 38:1–15.

20. Job 1:1–5.

21. Job 2:1–13.

22. Job 3:11–26.

23. Job 4:1–6.

24. Job 5:1–27.

25. Job 7:1–21.

26. Job 42:1–6, 10–17.

# TWO

# Greece

## INTRODUCTION

The earliest Greek literary works that have come down to us are *The Iliad* and *The Odyssey*, traditionally ascribed to Homer, who probably lived between c. 750 and c. 650 BCE. While the historical setting of these epic poems is the Trojan War, which the Greeks dated to about 1200 BCE, it is widely held that much of the social and cultural backdrop is the "dark age" that followed (c. 1200–c. 800 BCE). In the Homeric epics the gods play an active role in every area of life, including health and sickness. Apollo sends arrows that cause disease and death [2.1], and daimones (unseen supernatural powers) cause them as well (*Odyssey* 5.394–97). On the ritual level, the early Greeks regarded disease as retributive, the result of having offended a god or violated a sacred taboo [2.6]. Only after the offense was removed, the community purified, and the gods propitiated would the disease be eliminated. Hesiod, an epic poet who was perhaps a late contemporary of Homer, offered an alternative explanation on the mythological level. Diseases are daimones that escaped from Pandora's box and moved of their own accord throughout the world [2.2].

In everyday practice, Greeks could seek healing of supernaturally caused diseases from *iatromanteis*, shamans who traveled from city to city and purified communities from divine pollution [2.5]. For example, in the early sixth century BCE the Cretan Epimenides purified Athens, thus ending a plague that had fallen on the city because a magistrate had committed a sacrilege when he killed several men who had taken sanctuary in an Athenian temple [2.4]. But the Homeric epics speak also of an empirical approach to medicine. According to *The Odyssey* there existed a group called *demiourgoi*, who were itinerant members of a medical craft. They relied on their experience and skill to treat wounds, broken bones, and diseases symptomatically by employing traditional treatments that were passed on through apprenticeship. In the sixth century BCE groups of physicians began to assemble in several cities throughout the Mediterranean. While they did not train other physicians, they offered apprenticeships to aspiring doctors. Associated with one of the best known of these medical communities, Cos off the coast of Asia Minor, was the physician Hippocrates (c. 460–c. 380 BCE). Although he acquired a reputation as the "Father of Medicine," little is known about him. There exist only two contemporary references to Hippocrates (both by Plato), but he became the subject of several idealized legends after his death.

In the fifth century BCE Greek medicine began to develop beyond mere craftsmanship into an art with a body of theoretical knowledge. The craftsman or empiric was often skilled in practical knowledge and the application of traditional methods. But it was the addition of theory to practice that created learned medicine. The physician (*iatros*) attempted to understand disease and its causes in terms of natural processes [2.6]. To do so he turned to philosophy, from which he borrowed the ability to frame universal formulations and to forecast the course of illnesses [2.7, 2.8, 2.10]. The Hippocratic corpus was the earliest attempt to provide a theoretical basis for medicine. The collection consists of about seventy treatises, most of which were written in the fifth and fourth centuries BCE. The treatises eschew magical or divine factors in accounting for disease, in their place employing naturalistic theories of disease that were taken from pre-Socratic philosophers [2.6, 2.8]. The best known is the theory of the four humors, which was formulated by Empedocles (fl. 444–441 BCE) [2.10]. The writer of *On the Sacred Disease* argues that epilepsy, commonly attributed to divine possession, is not more sacred than any other disease, but has a natural cause [2.7]: "There is no need to put the disease in a special class and to consider it more divine than the others; they are all divine and all human. Each has a nature and power of its own; none is hopeless or incapable of treatment." While the Hippocratic treatises generally espouse a naturalistic explanation of disease [2.9], there is no evidence that their approach was regarded as atheistic. Hippocratic writers regarded nature as divine and medicine as a gift of the gods. Nor did they reject appeals to the gods for healing. "Prayer indeed is good, but while calling on the gods a man should himself lend a hand" (*Decorum* 87). But the introduction of professional medicine produced a standard of ethical behavior in the practice that is found in several

Hippocratic treatises and most famously summarized in the Hippocratic Oath [2.12].

Hippocratic medicine spread rapidly in the late fifth and fourth centuries BCE. But alongside this theoretical or speculative medicine, which assumed natural causes of illness and sought to heal by natural means, there remained a tradition of religious healing. Those suffering from illness sought divine healing from gods, demigods, and heroes. Initially cures were sought at the temple of any god or at the shrines of local heroes. But in the fifth century, Asklepios (*Latin*, Asclepius) emerged as the chief healing deity of Greece. In *The Iliad*, Asklepios is the "blameless physician" to whom the centaur Chiron teaches medicine. He is said in a later legend to have been a god. His cult initially came from Tricca in Thessaly (in northern Greece), but it spread to Epidaurus in the Peloponnese, which became the most important center of Asklepios's cult. It was carried throughout the Mediterranean world to Athens, to Pergamum in Asia Minor, to Crete, to Cyrene in North Africa, and finally in 291 BCE to Rome, where the god was worshiped as Aesculapius.

The temples of Asklepios (called *asklepieia*) attracted large numbers of sick people, who sought healing or an oracle in a dream. At Epidaurus those seeking healing underwent a ritual purification before offering simple sacrifices of cakes or fruit. The focal point of the pilgrimage was incubation, in which pilgrims spent a night in the *abaton*, which was the center of the temple [2.14]. In Epidaurus the abaton was a separate building near the actual temple—not just an incubation hall within the temple. Lying on a couch, the pilgrim would await a dream or vision from the god, who appeared holding a staff around which a snake was coiled, the caduceus, which would become a symbol of modern medical healing. The healing process varied to suit the pilgrim. Asklepios might merely touch the patient, or he might perform surgery or administer a healing drug in a dream. Sometimes a serpent or dog would bring healing by licking the wound. Whatever the means, when the incubants awoke the next morning, they expected to have been healed.

That many were cured of their illnesses or physical disabilities is evident from the several tablets, called *iamata*, that were inscribed at the temple site at Epidaurus, which recorded what are apparently case histories of pilgrims who had been healed [2.14]. On the one hand they follow a miracle narrative pattern, while on the other there are events that are medically plausible. These testimonials were doubtless meant to encourage pilgrims to trust that they too might experience the god's favor. The account of a woman who delivered a baby that she thought she had carried for five years, which is the opening story of the iamata, is the most wondrous of all. At this distance in time, it is impossible fully to explain how pilgrims were healed. General rationalistic approaches are simplistic. Perhaps many of the pilgrims suffered from chronic diseases that doctors could not successfully treat. Others probably suffered from conditions that were susceptible to a placebo effect. The *asklepieion* at Epidaurus grew over time to become a complex of buildings that included guesthouses for pilgrims, gymnasiums, theaters, stadiums, and baths, all of which created a sanatorium-like setting that offered a peaceful retreat and a therapeutic environment for physical healing and recuperation.

Asklepios was both the dispenser of divine healing through incubation and the patron of physicians. Galen (c. 129–c. 216 CE), a great physician and philosopher, referred to himself as a servant of Asklepios, who had healed him when Galen had a life-threatening abscess. Physicians did not doubt the god's ability to heal in any way he wished, whether miraculously or by natural means. They viewed religious healing as complementary to medicine. When they could offer no further medical help to their patients they had no objection to their seeking supernatural healing at the shrine of Asklepios. Since he was their patron, who blessed their efforts as medical practitioners, physicians saw no conflict with his healing in temples. They regarded both secular and temple medicine as legitimate means of healing, and indeed they existed in relative harmony but probably with little contact. The rapid spread of the cult of Asklepios in the fourth century BCE coincided with the decline of the older civic religions and appealed to the growing individualism of Greek religion. He was regarded as the most philanthropic of the gods and had an appeal for ordinary individuals that the great Olympian deities lacked. The poor, who could not afford physicians' fees, sought treatment at his temples. So popular was the worship of Asklepios that some seven hundred temples and shrines were devoted to his worship in the Greco-Roman world.

Following the conquest of the Persian Empire by Alexander the Great (who ruled 336–323 BCE), the beliefs and practices of foreign cults poured into Greece from Egypt and Asia, brought back by soldiers and traders returning from Alexander's campaigns. The Greek world was enlarged throughout the eastern Mediterranean, including the Hellenistic kingdoms of Macedonia, Egypt, and the vast Seleucid Empire in Asia. The cults' "mystery religions," as they have been called, offered a sense of personal union with the deity that was often formalized in a rite of initiation. They became enormously popular and, during the Hellenistic age (323–30 BCE), came to supplement the official cults that were maintained by the Greek city-states as the focal points of public worship. Many of them, such as Sarapis (Latin, Serapis), offered healing [2.15], which adherents of almost any Greek or foreign deity, demigod, or hero might expect of their religion. Incubation was the most common means of temple healing, but other forms existed as well. The use of magical practices in Greek medicine, common in Homeric and archaic Greece, did not play a major role in medical treatment. While some physicians might have resorted to incantations, amulets, or sympathetic magic, in general magical practices were the preserve of magicians, not of physicians. Indeed Greek medicine differed significantly in that regard from Mesopotamian and Egyptian medicine.

## TEXTS

---

### 2.1
### The plague of Troy
Homer, *The Iliad*[1]

*Greek literature begins with Homer, the traditional author of* The Iliad *and* The Odyssey. The Iliad *describes the epic war that was fought for ten years between the Achaean Greeks and the Trojans over Helen, the wife of Menelaus of Sparta, who had eloped with Paris, prince of Troy. It opens with a plague occasioned by the refusal of Agamemnon, leader of the Achaeans, to allow Chryses, priest of Apollo, to ransom his daughter Chryseis, whom Agamemnon has claimed as a spoil of war. Chryses prays to Apollo to strike the Achaeans with a plague. Apollo responds by attacking the Greek camp with disease-bearing arrows. As the plague takes a heavy toll, Achilles calls on the Achaeans to seek its cause. The seer Calchas names Agamemnon as the cause, and Agamemnon reluctantly agrees to give up Chryses but demands in her place Achilles's spoil Briseis, whom Achilles reluctantly agrees to surrender. Chryses, now satisfied, prays to Apollo to end the plague, which he does. But Achilles swears that he will no longer participate in the fighting, and the wrath of Achilles becomes a subplot in the narrative.*

*The plague with which* The Iliad *begins is perhaps the best-known example of the Greek belief that epidemics and diseases were retributive and that they were sent by the gods as reprisal for the failure of a city or even a single person to honor a god or fulfill a vow. The act of one man (in this case, Agamemnon) could result in his whole community's suffering. Plague was often regarded as the result of the anger of the gods, whose wrath needed to be propitiated.*

The wrath sing, goddess, of Peleus' son Achilles, the accursed wrath which brought countless sorrows upon the Achaeans, and sent down to Hades many valiant souls of warriors, and made the men themselves to be the spoil for dogs and birds of every kind; and thus the will of Zeus was brought to fulfillment. Of this sing from the time when first there parted in strife Atreus' son, lord of men, and noble Achilles.

Who then of the gods was it that brought these two together to contend? The son of Leto and Zeus; for he, angered at the king, roused throughout the army an evil pestilence, and the men were perishing, because to Chryses his priest the son of Atreus had done dishonor. For he had come to the swift ships of the Achaeans to free his daughter and he brought with him ransom past counting; and in his hands he held the ribbons of Apollo, who strikes from afar, on a staff of gold, and he implored all the Achaeans, but most of all the two sons of Atreus, the marshalers of armies: "Sons of Atreus, and you other well-greaved Achaeans, to you may the gods who have dwellings on Olympus grant that you sack the city of Priam, and return home safely; but set my dear child free for me, and accept the ransom in reverence for the son of Zeus, Apollo, who strikes from afar."

Then all the rest of the Achaeans shouted their agreement, to respect the priest and accept the glorious ransom; yet this did not please the heart of Agamemnon, son of Atreus, but he sent him away harshly, and laid on him a stern command: "Let me not find you, old man, by the hollow ships, either loitering now or coming back later, for fear your staff and the god's ribbon not protect you. But her I will not set free; before that, old age will come on her in our house, in Argos, far from her country, as she walks back and forth in front of the loom and shares my bed. But go; do not anger me, so that you may go the safer."

So he spoke, and the old man was seized with fear and obeyed his words. He went in silence along the shore of the loud-resounding sea; and then, when he had gone apart, the old man prayed earnestly to the lord Apollo, whom fair-haired Leto bore: "Hear me, you of the silver bow, who have under your protection Chryses and sacred Cilla, and who rule mightily over Tenedos, Smintheus, if ever I roofed over a pleasing shrine for you, or if ever I burned to you fat thigh pieces of bulls or goats, fulfill for me this wish: let the Danaans pay for my tears by your arrows."

So he spoke in prayer, and Phoebus Apollo heard him. Down from the peaks of Olympus he strode, angry at heart, with his bow and covered quiver on his shoulders. The arrows rattled on the shoulders of the angry god as he moved; and his coming was like the night. Then he sat down apart from the ships and let fly an arrow; terrible was the twang of the silver bow. The mules he attacked first and the swift dogs, but then on the men themselves he let fly his stinging arrows, and struck; and ever did the pyres of the dead burn thick.

For nine days the missiles of the god ranged through the army, but on the tenth Achilles called the army to the place of assembly, for the goddess, white-armed Hera, had put it in his heart; for she pitied the Danaans because she saw them dying. So, when they were assembled and met together, among them rose and spoke Achilles, swift of foot: "Son of Atreus, now I think we shall be driven back and return home, our plans thwarted—if we should escape death, that is—if indeed war and pestilence alike are to subdue the Achaeans. But come, let us ask some seer or priest, or some reader of dreams—for a dream too is from Zeus—who might tell us why Phoebus Apollo has conceived such anger, whether it is because of a vow that he blames us, or a hecatomb; in hope that perhaps he may accept the savor of lambs and unblemished goats, and be minded to ward off destruction from us."

When he had thus spoken he sat down, and among them rose up Calchas, son of Thestor, far the best of diviners, who had knowledge of all things that were, and that were to be, and that had been before, and who had guided the ships of the Achaeans to Ilios by the gift of prophecy that Phoebus Apollo had granted him. He with good intent addressed their assembly and spoke among them: "Achilles, dear to Zeus, you ask me to declare the wrath of Apollo, who smites from afar. Well, then, I will speak; but do you consider, and swear that you will be eager to defend me with word and hand; for in truth I think I shall anger a man who rules mightily over all the Argives, and whom the Achaeans obey. For a king is mightier when he is angry at a lesser man. For even if he swallows down his anger for the one day, still afterwards he holds resentment in his heart until he fulfills it. Consider, then, if you will keep me safe."

Then in answer to him spoke Achilles, swift of foot: "Take heart, and speak out any oracle you know, for by Apollo, dear to Zeus, to whom you pray,

Calchas, and declare oracles to the Danaans, no one, while I live and have sight on the earth, shall lay heavy hands on you beside the hollow ships, no one of all the Danaans, not even if it is Agamemnon you mean, who now declares himself far the best of the Achaeans."

Then the incomparable seer took heart, and spoke, saying: "It is not because of a vow that he blames us, nor a hecatomb, but because of the priest whom Agamemnon dishonored, and did not release his daughter nor accept the ransom. For this reason the god who strikes from afar has given woes, and will continue to give them, nor will he drive off from the Danaans loathsome destruction until we give back to her father the bright-eyed maiden, unbought, unransomed, and take a holy hecatomb to Chryses; then perhaps we might appease his wrath and persuade him."

## 2.2
## Pandora's gift
### Hesiod, *Works and Days*[2]

*Hesiod's (c. 700–c. 650 BCE)* Works and Days *is a didactic poem, a kind of almanac that provided advice to farmers laboring on their shrunken plots in poverty-stricken Boeotia, where he lived. Hesiod incorporated several myths into his poem, the best known being that of Pandora. After Prometheus stole fire from heaven, Zeus punished him by ordering Hephaestus to create the first woman, whose purpose was to sow confusion in the human race of men. She was called Pandora ("All Gifts") because she carried in a jar the many evils that had been given her as gifts by the gods. In spite of Prometheus's warning, his brother Epimetheus married Pandora, who opened the jar and released evils into the world, which had not previously existed and which spread confusion everywhere on land and sea. These evils included disease, which wandered randomly among humans. Hence it was the first woman who was blamed for the introduction of evil into the world.*

Straightway the famous Lame God moulded from the earth a likeness of a modest girl, on the plans of the son of Cronos. And grey-eyed Athene clothed the girl and adorned her, and the divine Graces and lady Persuasion put golden necklaces on her, and the fair-tressed Seasons crowned her with spring flowers. And Pallas Athene adorned her in every way. And the Slayer of Argus, the guide, put lies and crafty words and a deceitful Character in her breast according to the plans of Zeus the thunderer: and the herald of the gods put speech in her. And he named this woman Pandora, because all those who lived on Olympus gave her a gift, a bane for men who eat bread.

And when he had completed the sheer, hopeless snare, the father sent the famous Argus-Slayer, the swift messenger of the gods, to take it to Epimetheus as a gift. And Epimetheus did not think of what Prometheus had told him, namely not to receive a gift from Olympian Zeus, but to send it back, lest it prove an evil for mortals. But he took the gift, and only then realized that it was evil.

For before this the tribes of men lived on earth free from evils and hard toil and grievous diseases, which bring the Fates on men: for mortals grow old swiftly in misery. But the woman took off the great lid of the jar with her hands and scattered dire sorrows for men. Only Hope remained there within in an unbreakable home under the rim of the jar and did not fly out of the door. For before that the lid of the jar stopped her, by the designs of Zeus the cloud-gatherer who wields the aegis. But the other countless miseries wander among men. The earth is full of evils and the sea is full. Some diseases come upon men by day and some by night; they roam of their own free will, bringing evils to mortals, silently, for wise Zeus took away speech from them. Thus there is no way to escape the will of Zeus.

## 2.3
## The rewards of justice and injustice
### Hesiod, *Works and Days*[3]

*In Homer, the plague of Troy was sent by Apollo in retribution for an affront to his priest. In Hesiod, it was Pandora who introduced disease into the world. In the* Works and Days *Hesiod also propounded a theodicy, a vindication of divine goodness based on justice (dikē), when he wrote that Zeus rewarded justice with health, peace, and prosperity and that he punished those who practiced injustice (violence and evil deeds) with disease, famine, and poverty. An entire city sometimes suffered because it was punished for the actions of one wicked man who committed violence or exhibited hubris (overweening pride).*

But they who give straight judgments to strangers and to the men of the land, and who do not go astray from what is just, their city flourishes and the people prosper in it. Peace, the nurse of children, is abroad in their land, and all-seeing Zeus never decrees cruel war against them. Neither famine nor disaster ever haunt men who do true justice, but in good cheer they tend the fields they care for. The earth bears them an abundant livelihood, and on the mountains the oaks bear acorns on their tops and bees in their midst. Their woolly sheep are laden with fleeces: their women bear children like their parents. They flourish continually with good things and do not travel on ships, for the grain-giving earth bears them fruit.

But for those who practice evil violence and wicked deeds, for them the far-seeing son of Cronos decrees a penalty. Often a whole city suffers on account of a bad man who sins and contrives evil deeds. On them the son of Cronos brings great bane, both famine and plague down from heaven. And the people waste away and their women do not bear children, and the houses decline, through the plans of Olympian Zeus. Again at another time the son of Cronos either destroys their broad army, or their walls, or demolishes their ships on the sea.

## 2.4
### Epimenides's purification of Athens
Diogenes Laertius, *Lives of Eminent Philosophers: Epimenides*[4]

*In c. 632 BCE an Athenian nobleman and two-time Olympic victor, Cylon, seized the acropolis of Athens in an attempt to make himself a tyrant. He in turn was besieged by the Athenians at the order of the magistrate Megacles. Cylon escaped, and his men sought sanctuary in the temples. Contrary to sacred law, Megacles ordered the suppliants to be put to death. This act brought* miasma *(pollution) on the city and a plague. On the order of the Delphic oracle, Epimenides of Crete was summoned to purify the city and to remove the curse placed on it; the rite included offering two young men as a sacrifice. Epimenides was a semilegendary* iatromantis *(shaman), wonder-worker, and religious teacher about whom many stories arose: that he slept for fifty-seven years, that he wandered out of his body, that he died at a great age (157 or 299). This episode is informed by another religious explanation of disease offered by the Greeks: it is the result of pollution brought on a city for an evil deed.*

Then when the Athenians were attacked by plague, the Pythian priestess commanded them to purify the city. They sent a ship commanded by Nicias the son of Niceratus to Crete, to summon Epimenides. And he came in the forty-sixth Olympiad and purified the city and stopped the plague in the following way. He took sheep, some black, some white, and brought them to the Areopagus. There he let them loose to go wherever they liked, and he told men to follow them, and wherever each one lay down, to sacrifice to the local god. And thus the evil was stopped. And so even today one may find anonymous altars in different Athenian demes, which are memorials of the atonement. But some say that he declared the cause of the plague to be the pollution that Cylon brought and showed how to remove it: and in consequence two young men, Cratinus and Ctesibis, were put to death and the city was delivered from disaster.

He is said to have been the first to purify houses and fields and to establish temples. Some say that he did not go to sleep but withdrew himself for a period engaged in collecting roots.

## 2.5
## Empedocles, wonder-worker and healer

*Empedocles (fl. 444–441 BCE) was an iatromantis, wonder-worker, healer, orator, and statesman. He came from a distinguished aristocratic family in the Sicilian city of Acragas. He claimed to be a god and to be able to control winds and rain, to bring drought, and even to call the dead back to life. He was clearly an authoritative personality, and it is not surprising that he was offered the kingship of his city. He was also a physician who, according to Galen, founded a school of doctors in Italy or Sicily. His best-known contribution to medical theory was the theory of the four humors, which came to dominate Greek theoretical medicine. But he mixed naturalistic medicine with miracle working, as did other iatromanteis. Thus while he prescribed drugs (pharmaka), he also dispensed charms and spells. More than that, he gave prophecies and advertised himself as a purifier of pollution. As a pre-Socratic philosopher, he profoundly influenced subsequent Greek philosophy.*

### Empedocles and Clement[5]

Friends, who live in the great city of the yellow Acragas, up on the heights of the citadel, caring for good deeds, I give you greetings. An immortal god, mortal no more, I go about honoured by all, as is fitting, crowned with ribbons and fresh garlands; and by all whom I come upon as I enter their prospering towns, by men and women, I am revered. They follow me in their thousands, asking where lies the road to profit, some desiring prophecies, while others ask to hear the word of healing for every kind of illness, long transfixed by harsh pains.

### Empedocles[6]

You shall learn all the remedies that there are for ills and defence against old age, since for you alone will I accomplish all this. And you shall stay the force of the unwearied winds which sweep over the earth and lay waste the fields with their blasts; and then, if you wish, you shall bring back breezes in requital. After black rain you shall cause drought for men in due season, and then after summer drought cause air-inhabiting tree-nourishing streams. And you shall bring from Hades the strength of a dead man.

## 2.6
## The Scythian disease

*We are fortunate on occasion to have two very different explanations in Greek sources for the cause of an illness. Anarieis (impotence) was a condition that beset the Scythians, a nomadic race of Indo-European descent who occupied the Russian steppe in what is today Ukraine. The Scythians were famous for their cavalries of archers. Herodotus recorded that they once robbed a temple of Venus at Ascalon, which brought divine retribution on those who had committed the sacrilege and on their descendants. In typical Herodotean fashion he did not give his own opinion, but merely told the story as he heard it.*

### Herodotus, *The Histories*[7]

The Scythians who robbed the temple at Ascalon were punished by the goddess with the infliction of what is called the "female disease," and their descendants still suffer from it. This is the reason the Scythians give for this mysterious complaint, and travelers to the country can see what it is like. The Scythians call those who suffer from it "Enarees."

### Hippocrates, *Airs, Waters, Places*[8]

*The anonymous writer of the Hippocratic treatise* Airs, Waters, Places *gave a naturalistic explanation that differed from the version above. Like the Hippocratic author of* On the Sacred Disease, *he believed that all diseases were divine and that none was more so than any other. He attributed the Scythians' impotence to their approach to curing the problems that resulted from their manner of horseback riding. The Scythians' usual cure, according to this writer, was to cut the veins behind their ears, which (unknown to the Scythians) were ostensibly connected to the seminal vessels; this cure, he supposed, induced their impotence. This writer's "diagnosis" was wholly spurious; the explanation has no basis in medical fact.*

Moreover, the great majority among the Scythians become impotent, do women's work, live like women and converse accordingly. Such men they call "Anaries." Now the natives put the blame on to Heaven, and respect and worship these creatures, each fearing for himself. I too think these diseases are divine, and so are all others, no one being more divine or more human than any other; all are alike, and all divine. Each of them has a nature of its own, and none arises without its natural cause. How, in my opinion, this disease arises I will explain. The habit of riding causes swellings at the joints, because they are always astride their horses; in severe cases follow lameness and sores on the hips. They cure themselves in the following way. At the beginning of the disease they cut the vein behind each ear. When the blood has ceased to flow faintness comes over them and they sleep. Afterward they get up, some cured some not. Now, in my opinion, by this treatment the seed is destroyed. For by the side of the ear are veins, to cut which causes impotence, and I believe that these are the veins which they cut. After this treatment, when the Scythians approach a woman but cannot have intercourse, at first they take no notice and think no more about it. But when two, three or even more attempts are attended with no better success, thinking that they have sinned against Heaven they attribute thereto the cause, and put on woman's clothes, holding that they have lost their manhood. So they play the woman, and with the women do the same work as women do.

This affliction affects the rich Scythians because of their riding, not the lower classes but the upper, who possess the most strength; the poor, who do not ride, suffer less. But, if we suppose this disease to be more divine than any other, it ought to have attacked, not the highest richest classes only of the Scythians, but all classes equally—or rather the poor especially, if indeed the gods are pleased to receive from men respect and worship, and repay these with favours. For naturally the rich, having great wealth, make many sacrifices to the gods, and offer many votive offerings, and honour them, all of which things the poor, owing to their poverty, are less able to do; besides, they blame the gods for not giving them wealth, so that the penalties for such sins are likely to be paid by the poor rather than the rich. But the truth is, as I said above, these afflictions are neither more nor less divine than any others, and all and each are natural.

## 2.7
## The sacred disease
### Hippocrates, *On the Sacred Disease*[9]

*Epilepsy was popularly regarded in the Greek world as a sacred disease because its symptoms seemed to bear the marks of supernatural causes. Hence it was not treated by physicians but by purifiers and practitioners of magic and exorcism, all of whom in a sarcastic manner the writer of this text attacks as imposters. This Hippocratic treatise probably dates from the fifth century BCE, and its tone is both polemical and rhetorical. The author argues that the disease "comes from the same causes as other, from the things that come to and go from the body, from cold, sun, and from the changing restlessness of winds." These are the views of pre-Socratic philosophers, who provided the theories that undergirded medical naturalism, and indeed in many respects it echoes the language of* Airs, Waters, Places. *The writer argues that like other diseases epilepsy must be treated medically, and an experienced physician knows precisely which regimen will be effective. At this time, religious and supernatural causes of disease had been replaced by naturalistic explanations, which would hereafter characterize Greek secular medicine.*

5. But this disease [epilepsy] is in my opinion no more divine than any other; it has the same nature as other diseases, and the cause that gives rise to individual diseases. It is also curable, no less than other illnesses, unless by long lapse of time it be so ingrained as to be more powerful than the remedies that are applied. Its origin, like that of other diseases, lies in heredity. For if a phlegmatic parent has a phlegmatic child, a bilious parent a bilious child, a consumptive parent a consumptive child, and a splenetic parent a splenetic child, there is nothing to prevent some of the children suffering from this disease when one or the other of the parents suffered from it; for the seed comes from every part of the body, healthy seed from the healthy parts, diseased seed from the diseased parts. Another strong proof that this disease is no more divine than any other is that it affects the naturally phlegmatic, but does not attack the bilious. Yet, if it were more divine than others, this disease ought to have attacked all equally, without making any difference between bilious and phlegmatic.

. . .

21. This disease styled sacred comes from the same causes as other, from the things that come to and go from the body, from cold, sun, and from the changing restlessness of winds. These things are divine. So that there is no need to put the disease in a special class and to consider it more divine than the others; they are all divine and all human. Each has a nature and power of its own; none is hopeless or incapable of treatment. Most are cured by the same things as caused them. One thing is food for one thing, and another for another, though occasionally it does it harm. So the physician must know how, by distinguishing the seasons for individual things, he may assign to one thing nutriment and growth, and to another diminution and harm. For in this disease as in all others it is necessary, not to increase the illness, but to wear it down by allying to each what is most hostile to it, not that to which it is accustomed. For what is customary gives vigour and increase; what is hostile causes weakness and decay. Whoever knows how to cause in men by regimen moist or dry, hot or cold, he can cure this disease also, if he distinguish the seasons for useful treatment, without having recourse to purifications and magic.

### 2.8
### Prognosis
Hippocrates, *Prognostic*[10]

*Pronoia, or forecasting the course of an illness, was basic to Greek medicine. Pronoia included prognosis but went beyond it. It signified knowing something about a patient without being told. In fact, prognosis in this larger sense was of greater importance to the Greek physician than was diagnosis. Its significance is clearly explained in the text below. Its accuracy would build confidence in the patient, who needed grounds for trusting the attending physician. And it was essential for the physician to know the outcome of the disease from examining the symptoms and, above all, to know whether the patient would live or die. Hence the accuracy of his prognoses established the physician's credibility in a society in which there were no medical schools, no formal training beyond apprenticeship, and no license required to practice. Trust in the physician was the only basis of professional confidence. By predicting that the illness would lead to death, the physician was relieved of blame if the patient died.*

I hold that it is an excellent thing for a physician to practice forecasting. For if he discover and declare unaided by the side of his patients the present, the past and the future, and fill in the gaps in the account given by the sick, he will be the more believed to understand cases, so that men will confidently entrust themselves to him for treatment. Furthermore, he will carry out the treatment best if he know beforehand from the present symptoms what will take place later. Now to restore every patient to health is impossible. To do so indeed would have been better even than forecasting the future. But as a matter of fact men do die, some owing to the severity of the disease before they summon the physician, others expiring immediately after calling him in—living one day or a little longer—before the physician by his art can combat each disease. It is necessary, therefore, to learn the natures of such diseases, how much they exceed the strength of men's bodies, and to learn how to forecast them. For in this way you will justly win respect and be an able physician. For the longer time you plan to meet each emergency the greater your power to save those who have a chance of recovery, while you will be blameless if you learn and declare beforehand those who will die and those who will get better.

## 2.9
## Clinical records
### Hippocrates, *Epidemics I: Fourteen Cases*[11]

*Closely related to the development of prognosis in Greek medicine were the forty-two case histories that are in the Hippocratic corpus. The clinical notes preserved in* Epidemics *seem to be a physician's daybook in which the symptoms were recorded based on meticulous observation. These notes aided physicians in recognizing and forecasting the course of diseases that they might have had to treat. In reading about Silenus (case 2) and the woman by the shore (case 13) one is struck by the detailed clinical observation and professional distance of the physician. The symptoms are described succinctly and objectively and without any attempt at prognosis or diagnosis. By the time a practitioner was called in, all patients were severely ill, and in most cases they died.*

### Case 2

Silenus lived on Broadway near the place of Eualcidas. After overexertion, drinking, and exercises at the wrong time he was attacked by fever. He began by having pains in the loins, with heaviness in the head and tightness of the neck. From the bowels on the first day there passed copious discharges of bilious matter, unmixed, frothy, and highly coloured. Urine black, with a black sediment; thirst; tongue dry; no sleep at night.

*Second day.* Acute fever, stool more copious, thinner, frothy; urine black; uncomfortable night; slightly out of his mind.

*Third day.* General exacerbation; oblong tightness of the hypochondrium, soft underneath, extending on both sides to the navel; stools thin, blackish; urine turbid, blackish; no sleep at night; much rambling, laughter, singing; no power of restraining himself.

*Fourth day.* Same symptoms.

*Fifth day.* Stools unmixed, bilious, smooth, greasy; urine thin, transparent; lucid intervals.

*Sixth day.* Slight sweats about the head; extremities cold and livid; much tossing; nothing passed from the bowels; urine suppressed; acute fever.

*Seventh day.* Speechless; extremities would no longer get warm; no urine.

*Eighth day.* Cold sweat all over; red spots with sweat, round, small like acne, which persisted without subsiding. From the bowels with slight stimulus there came a copious discharge of solid stools, thin, as it were unconcocted, painful. Urine painful and irritating. Extremities grow a little warmer; fitful sleep; coma; speechlessness; thin, transparent urine.

*Ninth day.* Same symptoms.

*Tenth day.* Took no drink; coma; fitful sleep. Discharges from the bowels similar; had a copious discharge of thickish urine, which on standing left a farinaceous, white deposit, extremities again cold.

*Eleventh day.* Death.

From the beginning the breath in this case was throughout rare and large. Continuous throbbing of the hypochondrium; age about twenty.

## Case 13

A woman lying sick by the shore, who was three months gone with child, was seized with fever, and immediately began to feel pains in the loins.

*Third day.* Pain in the neck and in the head, and in the region of the right collar-bone. Quickly she lost her power of speech, the right arm was paralyzed, with a convulsion, after the manner of a stroke; completely delirious. An uncomfortable night, without sleep; bowels disordered with bilious, unmixed, scanty stools.

*Fourth day.* Her speech was recovered, but was indistinct; convulsions; pains in the same parts remained; painful swelling in the hypochondrium; no sleep; utter delirium; bowels disordered; urine thin, and not of a good colour.

*Fifth day.* Acute fever; pain in the hypochondrium; utter delirium; bilious stools. At night sweated; was without fever.

*Sixth day.* Rational; general relief, but pain remained about the left collar-bone; thirst; urine thin; no sleep.

*Seventh day.* Trembling; some coma; slight delirium; pains in the region of the collar-bone and the left upper arm remained; other symptoms relieved; quite rational. For three days there was an intermission of fever.

*Eleventh day.* Relapse; rigor; attack of fever. But about the fourteenth day the patient vomited bilious, yellow matter fairly frequently; sweated; a crisis took off the fever.

## 2.10
### The humoral theory
Hippocrates, *On the Nature of Man*[12]

*The most widely accepted physiological theory in Greek medicine was the humoral theory of Empedocles, which was based on quaternaries, or groups of four. Just as there were four elements (earth, air, fire, and water), which produced four qualities (warmth, cold, dryness, and wetness), so there were four fluids (humors) in the body (blood, phlegm, yellow bile, and black bile). If these humors were in a state of harmony, they resulted in a healthy body. An imbalance of the humors produced disease. The aim of medical treatment was to prescribe a diet or regimen that would counterbalance the disease and restore the body to health. There were many variants of the theory, but what became the canonical humoral theory was the one adopted by Galen in the second century CE, and his authority established its supremacy over all others. Standard medical treatment was based on the humoral theory throughout the classical period and into the eighteenth century. The theory is described in the Hippocratic treatise excerpted below.*

4. The body of man has in itself blood, phlegm, yellow bile, and black bile; these make up the nature of his body, and through these he feels pain or enjoys health. Now he enjoys the most perfect health when these elements are duly proportioned to one another in respect of compounding, power

and bulk, and when they are perfectly mingled. Pain is felt when one of these elements is in defect or excess, or is isolated in the body without being compounded with all the others. For when an element is isolated and stands by itself, not only must the place which it left become diseased, but the place where it stands in a flood must, because of the excess, cause pain and distress. In fact, when more of an element flows out of the body than is necessary to get rid of superfluity, the emptying causes pain. If, on the other hand, it be to an inward part that there takes place the emptying, the shifting, and the separation from other elements, the man certainly must, according to what has been said, suffer from a double pain, one in the place left, and another in the place flooded.

5. Now I promised to show that what are according to me the constituents of man remain always the same, according to both convention and nature. These constituents are, I hold, blood, phlegm, yellow bile, and black bile. First I assert that the names of these according to convention are separated, and that none of them has the same name as the others; furthermore, that according to nature their essential forms are separated, phlegm being quite unlike blood, blood being quite unlike bile, bile being quite unlike phlegm. How could they be like one another, when their colors appear not alike to the sight nor does their touch seem alike to the hand? For they are not equally warm, nor cold, nor dry, nor moist. Since they are so different from one another in essential form and in power, they cannot be one, if fire and water are not one.

## 2.11
## The plague of Athens
Thucydides, *History of the Peloponnesian War*[13]

*Thucydides (c. 455–c. 400 BCE) was an Athenian general of aristocratic background and education who reported that he began writing his* History of the Peloponnesian War *shortly after it began. The war was waged between Athens and Sparta and their allies from 431 to 404 BCE. Although he lived until after the end of the war Thucydides never completed his* History, *but he gave us one of the most famous accounts of a plague in any ancient historian's work (for a modern example, see Daniel Defoe's* Journal of the Plague Year *[1722]). Doubtless, Thucydides was influenced by the opening pages of* The Iliad, *whose celebrated narrative of the plague sent by Apollo most of his readers knew well. He reported that he personally experienced the plague and recov-*

*ered and that he was therefore a reliable witness. But he gave the plague greater prominence in his narrative than was required in a history of a war. He described the symptoms in detail, perhaps influenced to some degree by the case studies in the Epidemics. He then used disease as a model for understanding history: just as a disease can be diagnosed and recognized when it recurs, so social ills recur in the body politic, and since human nature remains the same, the historian can help readers recognize them in the future. Here he applied pronoia (foreknowledge) in its medical sense to the study of history. Thucydides, moreover, viewed the plague not merely as a major factor in the decline of Athens but as a case study in mass psychology. He described the moral degradation of Athenians when faced with a breakdown of civil society and its religious constraints on extreme behavior.*

In this way the funeral was conducted in the winter that came at the end of the first year of the war. At the beginning of the following summer the Peloponnesians and their allies, with two-thirds of their total forces as before, invaded Attica, again under the command of the Spartan King Archidamus, the son of Zeuxidamus. Taking up their positions, they set about the devastation of the country.

They had not been many days in Attica before the plague first broke out among the Athenians. Previously attacks of the plague had been reported from many other places in the neighborhood of Lemnos and elsewhere, but there was no record of the disease being so virulent anywhere else or causing so many deaths as it did in Athens. At the beginning the doctors were quite incapable of treating the disease because of their ignorance of the right methods. In fact mortality among the doctors was the highest of all, since they came more frequently in contact with the sick. Nor was any other human art or science of any help at all. Equally useless were prayers made in the temples, consultation of oracles, and so forth; indeed, in the end people were so overcome by their sufferings that they paid no further attention to such things.

The plague originated, so they say, in Ethiopia in upper Egypt, and spread from there into Egypt itself and Libya and much of the territory of the King of Persia. In the city of Athens it appeared suddenly, and the first cases were among the population of Piraeus, where there were no wells at that time, so that it was supposed by them that the Peloponnesians had poisoned the reservoirs. Later, however, it appeared also in the upper city, and by this time the deaths were greatly increasing in number. As to the question of how it could have come about or what causes can be found adequate to explain its powerful effect on nature, I must leave that to be considered by other writers, with or without medical experience. I myself shall merely describe what it was like, and set down the symptoms, knowledge of which will enable it to be recognized, if it should ever break out again. I had the disease myself and saw others suffering from it.

That year, as is generally admitted, was particularly free from all other kinds of illness, though those who did not have any illness previously all caught the plague in the end. In other cases, however, there seemed to be no reason for the attacks. People in perfect health suddenly began to have burning feelings in the head; their eyes became red and inflamed; inside their mouths there was bleeding from the throat and tongue, and the breath became unnatural and unpleasant. The next symptoms were sneezing and hoarseness of voice, and before long the pain settled on the chest and was accompanied by coughing. Next the stomach was affected with stomach-aches and with vomitings of every kind of bile that has been given a name by the medical profession, all this being accompanied by great pain and difficulty. In most cases there were attacks of ineffectual retching, producing violent spasms; this sometimes ended with this stage of the disease, but sometimes continued long afterwards. Externally the body was not very hot to the touch, nor was there any pallor: the skin was rather reddish and livid, breaking out into small pustules and ulcers. But inside there was a feeling of burning, so that people could not bear the touch of even the lightest linen clothing, but wanted to be completely naked, and indeed most of all would have liked to plunge into cold water. Many of the sick who were uncared for actually did so, plunging into the water-tanks in an effort to relieve a thirst which was unquenchable; for it was just the same with them whether they drank much or little. Then all the time they were afflicted with insomnia and the desperate feeling of not being able to keep still.

In the period when the disease was at its height, the body, so far from wasting away, showed surprising powers of resistance to all the agony, so that there was still some strength left on the seventh or eighth day, which was the time when, in most cases, death came from the internal fever. But if people survived this critical period, then the disease descended to the bowels, producing violent ulcerations and uncontrollable diarrhoea, so that most of them died later as a result of the weakness caused by this. For the disease, first settling in the head, went on to affect every part of the body in turn, and even when people escaped its worst effects, it still left its traces on them by fastening upon the extremities of the body. It affected the genitals, the fingers, and the toes, and many of those who recovered lost the use of these members; some, too, went blind. There were also some who, when they first began to get better, suffered from a total loss of memory, not knowing who they were themselves and being unable to recognize their friends.

Words indeed fail one when one tries to give a general picture of this disease; and as for the sufferings of individuals, they seemed almost beyond the capacity of human nature to endure. Here in particular is a point where this plague showed itself to be something quite different from ordinary diseases: though there were many dead bodies lying about unburied, the birds and animals that eat human flesh either did not come near them or, if they did taste the flesh, died of it afterwards. Evidence for this may be found in the fact that there was a complete disappearance of all birds of prey: they were not to be seen either round the bodies or anywhere else. But dogs, being domestic animals, provided the best opportunity of observing this effect of the plague.

These, then, were the general features of the disease, though I have omitted all kinds of peculiarities which occurred in various individual cases. Meanwhile, during all this time there was no serious outbreak of any of the usual kinds of illness; if any such cases did occur, they ended in the plague. Some died in neglect, some in spite of every possible care being taken of them. As for a recognized method of treatment, it would be true to say that no such thing existed: what did good in some cases did harm in others. Those with naturally strong constitutions were no better able than the weak to resist the disease, which carried away all alike, even those who were treated and dieted with the greatest care. The most terrible thing of all was the despair into which people fell when they realized that they had caught the plague; for they would immediately adopt an attitude of utter hopelessness, and, by giving in in this way, would lose their powers of resistance. Terrible, too, was the sight of people dying like sheep through having caught the disease as a result of nursing others. This indeed caused more deaths than anything else. For when people were afraid to visit the sick, then they died with no one to look after them; indeed, there were many houses in which all the inhabitants perished through lack of any attention. When, on the other hand, they did visit the sick, they lost their own lives, and this was particularly true of those who made it a point of honour to act properly. Such people felt ashamed to think of their own safety and went into their friends' houses at times when even the members of the household were so overwhelmed by the weight of their calamities that they had actually given up the usual practice of making laments for the dead. Yet still the ones who felt most pity for the sick and the dying were those who had had the plague themselves and had recovered from it. They knew what it was like and at the same time felt themselves to be safe, for no one caught the disease twice, or, if he did, the second attack was never fatal. Such people were congratulated on all sides, and they themselves were so elated at the time of their recovery that they fondly imagined that they could never die of any other disease in the future.

A factor which made matters much worse than they were already was the removal of people from the country into the city, and this particularly affected the incomers. There were no houses for them, and, living as they did during the hot season in badly ventilated huts, they died like flies. The bodies of the dying were heaped one on top of the other, and half-dead creatures could be seen staggering about in the streets or flocking around the fountains in their desire for water. The temples in which they took up their quarters were full of the dead bodies of people who had died inside them. For the catastrophe was so overwhelming that men, not knowing what would happen next to them, became indifferent to every rule of religion or of law. All the funeral ceremonies which used to be observed were now disorganized, and they buried the dead as best they could. Many people, lacking the necessary means of burial because so many deaths had already occurred in their households, adopted the most shameless methods. They would arrive first at a funeral pyre that had been made by others, put their own dead upon it and set it alight; or, finding another pyre burning, they would throw the corpse that they were carrying on top of the other one and go away.

In other respects also Athens owed to the plague the beginnings of a state of unprecedented lawlessness. Seeing how quick and abrupt were the changes of fortune which came to the rich who suddenly died and to those who had previously been penniless but now inherited their wealth, people now began openly to venture on acts of self-indulgence which before then they used to keep dark. Thus they resolved to spend their money quickly and to spend it on pleasure, since money and life alike seemed equally ephemeral. As for what is called honour, no one showed himself willing to abide by its laws, so doubtful was it whether one would survive to enjoy the name for it. It was generally agreed that what was both honourable and valuable was the pleasure of the moment and everything that might conceivably contribute to that pleasure. No fear of god or law of man had a restraining influence. As for the gods, it seemed to be the same thing whether one worshipped them or not, when one saw the good and the bad dying indiscriminately. As for offences against human law, no one expected to live long enough to be brought to trial and punished: instead everyone felt that already a far heavier sentence had been passed on him and was hanging over him, and that before the time for its execution arrived it was only natural to get some pleasure out of life.

This, then, was the calamity which fell upon Athens, and the times were hard indeed, with men dying inside the city and the land being laid waste.

## 2.12
## The Hippocratic Oath[14]

*The first mention of the Hippocratic Oath comes from the first century CE and the Roman writer Scribonius Largus. It is preserved in the Hippocratic corpus, but its date is unknown and there is no evidence to connect it with Hippocrates. It begins with an invocation to the gods of healing. The invocation is followed by the covenant, which is a contract between the teacher and his pupil, who is adopted into the teacher's family as if he were one of his children. It establishes a mutual relationship within the extended family but keeps the teachings of his master within that family circle. The covenant is followed by the duties of the physician to those whom he treats. Three prohibitions (not to harm the sick, not to administer a deadly drug, and not to give abortifacients to women) are followed by the pledge "In purity and holiness I will guard my life and my art." There follow three additional prohibitions: to avoid the practice of surgery, to abstain from sexual intercourse with any member of the patient's household, and to not reveal secrets that are acquired in his practice. The last paragraph promises honor for the person who fulfills the oath and the opposite (dishonor) if he breaks it.*

*The call for purity and holiness, even if they refer to ritual purity, impart a religious tenor to the document as does the moralistic nature of the prohibitions. The oath prohibits certain procedures, such as abortion, euthanasia, and surgery, which were routinely practiced by Greek physicians and were not prohibited in the Hippocratic deontological treatises. These treatises deal with professional ethical obligations. Hence it has been argued by Ludwig Edelstein and others that the oath may have arisen among a restricted group of physicians, such as the Pythagoreans. We have no evidence that it was ever sworn in the classical world, but its religious and moral tone attracted the attention of early Christians and, later, Jews and Muslims, all of whom modified it to suit their own religious traditions.*

I swear by Apollo Physician and Asclepius and Hygieia and Panaceia and all the gods and goddesses, making them my witnesses, that I will fulfill according to my ability and judgment this oath and this covenant:

To hold him who has taught me this art as equal to my parents and to live my life in partnership with him, and if he is in need of money to give him a share of mine, and to regard his offspring as equal to my brothers in male lineage and to teach them this art—if they desire to learn it—without fee and covenant; to give a share of precepts and oral instruction and all the other learning to my sons and to the sons of him who has instructed me and to pupils who have signed the covenant and have taken an oath according to the medical law, but to no one else.

I will apply dietetic measures for the benefit of the sick according to my ability and judgment; I will keep them from harm and injustice.

I will neither give a deadly drug to anybody if asked for it, nor will I make a suggestion to this effect. Similarly I will not give to a woman an abortive remedy. In purity and holiness I will guard my life and my art.

I will not use the knife, not even on sufferers from stone, but will withdraw in favor of such men as are engaged in this work.

Whatever houses I may visit, I will come for the benefit of the sick, remaining free of all intentional injustice, of all mischief and in particular of sexual relations with both female and male persons, be they free or slaves.

What I may see or hear in the course of the treatment or even outside of the treatment in regard to the life of men, which on no account one must spread abroad, I will keep to myself holding such things shameful to be spoken about.

If I fulfill this oath and do not violate it, may it be granted to me to enjoy life and art, being honored with fame among all men for all time to come; if I transgress it and swear falsely, may the opposite of all this be my lot.

## 2.13
## An oath in the shrine of Agdistis
A. D. Nock, *Conversion*[15]

*The following text is not a medical oath, but it resembles the Hippocratic Oath in its religious tenor. It was found in a private shrine of the goddess Agdistis in Philadelphia in western Asia Minor and dates from the Hellenistic period, c. 100 BCE. Worshipers were required to swear an oath of purity, which was not merely about ritual purity but included moral purity. Purity was often required for entrance to a temple, such as that of Asklepios at Epidaurus. But that was a matter of ritual purity: a certain time period was required after intercourse or after contact with a corpse in order for the unholiness of the impure act to wear off. In this oath, right conduct or virtue is not an ethical standard sanctioned by philosophy but a matter of religious sanction.*

Let men and women, slave and free, when coming into this shrine swear by all the gods that they will not deliberately plan any evil guile, or baneful poison against any man or woman; that they will neither know nor use harmful spells; that they will neither turn to nor recommend to others nor have a hand in love-charms, abortives, contraceptives, or doing robbery or murder; that they will steal nothing but will be well-disposed to this house, and if any man does or purposes any of these things they will not keep silence but will reveal it and avenge. A man is not to have relations with the wife of another, whether a free woman or a married slave, or with a boy, or with a virgin, or to counsel this to another. . . . Let not woman or man who do the aforementioned acts come into this shrine; for in it are enthroned mighty deities, and they observe such offences and will not tolerate those who transgress their commands. . . . These commands were set up by the rule of Agdistis, the most holy guardian and mistress of this shrine. May she put good intentions in men and women, free and slave alike, that they may abide by what is here inscribed; and may all men and women who are confident of their uprightness touch this writing, which gives the commandments of the god, at the monthly and at the annual (?) sacrifices in order that it may be clear who abides by them and who does not. O Saviour Zeus, hear our words, and give us a good requital, health, deliverance, peace, safety on land and sea.

## 2.14
## Healings by Asklepios at Epidaurus
### Frederick C. Grant, *Hellenistic Religions*[16]

*Medical historians used to believe that temple healing in Greece was over time superseded by naturalistic healing as the society grew more rational in its thinking. In fact, temple healing first became popular in the last quarter of the fifth century BCE, at the same time that the Hippocratic treatises began to appear. The cult of Asklepios was centered in the small town of Epidaurus in the northwestern Peloponnese of Greece, where a temple was built to the god in the fourth century BCE, though his worship there may antedate the fourth century. The precinct of Asklepios became the most celebrated healing site in Greece, and for several centuries it attracted pilgrims who sought healing. It appealed not merely to the poor and uneducated, but to upper-class and educated Greeks as well. Asklepios's popularity did not, however, result in the decline of secular healing. There was a place in Greek society for both kinds of healing, which complemented each other. In his temples, Asklepios appeared to pilgrims in dreams, in which he sometimes performed surgery; at other times, he followed similar procedures to those that are described in the Hippocratic treatises, doing what an ordinary physician might do. But he did not always follow standard therapies, or he used them in different ways. Sometimes pilgrims awoke healed; on other occasions the god or his priests or physicians—for there were physicians that could be consulted in the temple—prescribed a healing regimen or drugs.*

*The priests often urged those who had been healed to post iamata (inscriptions) that testified to their divine healing. These were stories of success or of unbelievers, such as the man whose fingers were paralyzed (3) or Ambrosia from Athens (4), who came as doubters but left as believers in Asklepios's healing ability. Some of the testimonials are of clearly miraculous healings, such as that of Cleo, who had been pregnant for five years (1), or the blind man who received new eyes (9). Others, such as the dumb boy (5), suggest the impact of shock in curing an illness that we today would call psychosomatic. The account of Pandarus (6), while not impossible, defies rational explanation.*

### "God! Good fortune!"
#### *Healings of Apollo and Asklepios*

1. *Cleo was pregnant for five years.* When she had now been pregnant for five years, she turned for help to the god and slept in the holy of holies

[*abaton*]. As soon as she came out again and had left the sacred precincts she bore a son, who, as soon as he was born, washed himself at the spring and walked around with his mother. Having found such favor, she inscribed upon the gift offering:

It is not the greatness of the tablet that is wonderful, but the god!
Cleo bore for five years the burden beneath her heart,
Until she slept here, and the god made her well.

. . .

3. *A man whose fingers, all but one, were paralyzed.* He came to the god looking for help, but when he read the tablets set up in the temple he gave no credence to the healings and made fun of the inscriptions. But as he slept, he had the following dream. It seemed to him that he was playing dice in the temple and was about to make a throw. The god appeared to him, and sprang upon his hand and stretched out his fingers. Then he got up and, still in his dream, the man clenched his fist and opened it, stretching out one finger after another. After he had stretched them all out, the god asked him if he still refused to believe what the inscriptions related, and he said "No." "Well then," answered the god, "since you formerly refused to believe what is not unbelievable, you shall henceforth be known as 'the Doubter.'" When it was day, he came out cured.

4. *Ambrosia from Athens, who was blind in one eye.* She came to the god seeking help, but as she went about the temple she mocked at the many records of cures: "It is unbelievable and impossible that the lame and the blind can be made whole by merely dreaming!" But in her sleep she had a dream. It seemed to her that the god came up and promised to make her whole; only in return she must present a gift offering in the temple—a silver pig, in memory of her stupidity. After saying this he cut open her defective eye and poured in some drug. And when it was day, she went forth cured.

5. *A Dumb Boy.* He came to the sanctuary seeking to recover his voice. As he was presenting his first offering and performing the usual ceremony, the acolyte who bears the fire [for the sacrifice] to the god turned and said to the father of the boy, "Will you promise, if you get your wish, between now and the end of the year to bring the offering you owe as a fee for the healing?" At once the boy cried out, "I promise!" The father was greatly astonished, and told him to say it again. The boy said it again and was made whole from that moment.

6. *Pandarus a Thessalian, who had branded marks on his forehead.* He slept [in the sanctuary] and had the following dream. It seemed to him as if the god bound up the brand marks with a bandage and commanded him to take it with him when he left the holy of holies and place it in the temple. When it was day, he went out and took the bandage off, and he saw that his face was free from the marks. In the temple he dedicated the bandage, which had the branding marks transferred to it from his forehead.

7. *Echedorus received the branding marks of Pandarus in addition to his own.* This man had received money from Pandarus to present to the god here at Epidauros on his behalf, but he did not deliver it. In his sleep he had the following dream. He dreamt that the god came and stood over him and asked him if he had received certain money from Pandarus for an offering[?] to the temple. He replied that he had received nothing of the kind, but that if he would heal him he would set up a statue for him. Thereupon the god fastened upon him the bandage of Pandarus, which had covered the branding marks, and bade him to take it off when he had left the holy of holies, wash his face at the spring, and then look in the water. When it was day, he came out of the holy of holies and took off the bandage. The bandage no longer bore the brand marks. Instead, as he looked in the water, he saw that his face was marked not only with his own stigmata but also with the letters which once had been on Pandarus' forehead.

8. *Euphanes, a boy of Epidaurus.* This one was suffering from stone, and slept in the temple. And it seemed to him as if the god stood by him and said, "What will you give me if I make you well?" He replied, "Ten dice." Then the god laughed and promised to relieve his sufferings. When it was day, he came out cured.

9. *A man who was so blind that only the lids were left,* while the hollows of his eyes were completely empty, came seeking help from the god. Some of those who were present in the temple held forth on his stupidity in believing that he could ever see again, in spite of the fact that nothing was left of his eyes but only the empty sockets. But as he slept a vision came to him. He dreamed that the god prepared some drug, opened his eyelids, and poured it in. When day came, he came forth seeing with both eyes.

## 2.15
## The cult of Sarapis
Frederick C. Grant, *Hellenistic Religions*[17]

*Sarapis (Latin, Serapis) was an Egyptian god created by Ptolemy I of Egypt (283/2–246 BCE) to unite the Greeks and Egyptians in a common worship. The cult of Sarapis was spread by traders throughout the Mediterranean world to many cities, where he became identified with several Greek gods as a healer, a miracle worker, and (like Asklepios) a god who spoke in dreams. This text is a letter written to a man named Apollonios by Zoilos of Aspendos in 258/57 BCE. The writer was a person of considerable wealth and position (he sent the letter by way of the king's cousins), and the recipient was an acquaintance of King Ptolemy. Zoilos related that in a series of dreams the god Sarapis repeatedly appeared to him and commanded him to build a shrine with an altar for his worship near the harbor in Alexandria. When Zoilos delayed doing so, he was struck by a life-threatening illness. On recovery he delayed further in deliver-ing the message and suffered a relapse that lasted four months. In the letter, he begs Apollonios to undertake the building. Zoilos indicates that it will bring good health and fortune.*

To Apollonios, greetings from Zoilos of Aspendos . . . which the king's cous-ins will deliver to you. As I was worshiping the god Sarapis and interceding for your health and your favor with King Ptolemy, Sarapis repeatedly, in dreams, laid upon me the duty of going to you and conveying to you the fol-lowing directions: A Sarapieion and a sacred area must be built for him in the Greek quarter beside the harbor; a priest must be appointed and offer sacrifices there for us. When I begged him to release me from this duty, he let me fall into a severe illness, so that I was even in danger of my life. Then I prayed to him [and promised] that, if he would make me well, I should undertake the mission and carry out his command. Just when I had recov-ered, someone came from Cnidus and began building a Sarapieion at the place, and had ordered the stone brought there. Later on, the god forbade him to build, and he went away. When I came to Alexandria and hesitated to go to you with my message until you at last granted me the opportunity, I had a relapse that lasted for four months, and so I could not come to you im-mediately. Please, Apollonios, carry out the command of the god, so that Sarapis may be gracious to you and lead you to still greater influence with the king and [grant you] fame and physical health. You need not be alarmed over this commission and the large expenditure it entails; instead, it will be greatly to your advantage, for I will myself share in managing the whole undertaking. May all go well with you!

## NOTES

1. Homer, *Iliad*, vol. 1: *Books 1–12*, trans. A. T. Murray, rev. William F. Wyatt (Cambridge, MA: Harvard University Press, 1999), lines 1–100. Loeb Classical Library, vol. 170. Copyright © 1999 by the President and Fellows of Harvard College. Loeb Classical Library is a registered trademark of the President and Fellows of Harvard College.

2. Hesiod, *Works and Days* 70–105, in Geoffrey E. R. Lloyd, *In the Grip of Disease: Studies in the Greek Imagination* (Oxford: Oxford University Press, 2003), 33–35. Copyright © G. E. R. Lloyd 2003.

3. Hesiod, *Works and Days* 225–47, ibid., 35.

4. Diogenes Laertius 1:110, 112, ibid., 37.

5. Empedocles, frag. 112 (Diogenes Laertius 8.62.1–10; Clement, *Stromatis* 6.30. 9–11), ibid., 39.

6. Empedocles, frag. 111 (Diogenes Laertius 8.59), ibid.

7. Herodotus, *Histories* 1.105.4, ibid., 129.

8. Hippocrates, *Airs, Waters, Places* 22, ibid., 129.

9. Hippocrates, *On the Sacred Disease* 5.21, in Cohen and Drabkin, *Source Book in Greek Science*, 473–74.

10. Hippocrates, *Prognostic* 1, ibid., 498–99.

11. Hippocrates, *Epidemics* I, cases 2, 13, ibid., 492–93.

12. Hippocrates, *On the Nature of Man* 4–5, in *Hippocrates*, vol. 4, trans. W. H. S. Jones (Cambridge, MA: Harvard University Press, first published 1931). Loeb Classical Library, vol. 150. Loeb Classical Library is a registered trademark of the President and Fellows of Harvard College.

13. Thucydides, *History of the Peloponnesian War*, trans. Rex Warner, with an introduction and notes by M. I. Finley (London: Penguin Classics, 1954; rev. ed., 1972), 2.47.1–54. Translation copyright © Rex Warner, 1954. Introduction and appendices copyright © M. I. Finley, 1972. Reproduced by permission of Penguin Books Ltd.

14. Ludwig Edelstein, *The Hippocratic Oath: Text, Translation, and Interpretation* (Baltimore, MD: The Johns Hopkins Press, 1943). Copyright © 1943 The Johns Hopkins Press. Reprinted with permission of Johns Hopkins University Press.

15. Nock, *Conversion*, 217.

16. Grant, *Hellenistic Religions*, 56–58.

17. Ibid., 144–45.

# THREE

# *Rome*

## INTRODUCTION

Rome was, according to tradition, founded in 753 BCE. For the first six centuries of their history, the Romans claimed to have lived without either medicine or physicians. They used native folk remedies, which they supplemented with magic and divination that they inherited from the Etruscans [3.8]. The paterfamilias (the eldest male member of the household, which usually included slaves and up to three generations of lineal descendants) often administered folk remedies to his household. A well-known example of such a family practitioner was Cato the Elder (234–149 BCE) [3.6]. Cato relied on folk remedies together with prayers, sacrifices, magical incantations, and rituals to protect his family and farm [3.7]. He was renowned for his advocacy and use of cabbage in medicinal recipes and for his contempt for Greek medical theories and practitioners.

The earliest Roman religion was animistic. The early Romans worshiped spiritual powers without defined personalities, which they called numina [3.1]. Under the influence of the Etruscans, they came over time to represent numina as gods, many of whom they identified with Greek gods with similar characteristics, but animistic elements remained. Roman religion was a state cult, staffed by unpaid priests who carried out formal observances that maintained the *pax deorum* (protection of the gods) and guaranteed continuing divine favor toward the city and its fortunes. The Romans believed that if they neglected to observe formal religious obligations, the gods would send disasters. Hence public disasters like epidemics, droughts, and defeats in battle were explained as having been sent by the gods, and great care was taken to propitiate the gods to avert their anger

[3.2]. The earliest Romans had no specific gods associated with disease or healing, although certain deities might be appealed to if they were thought to be especially concerned with body parts or bodily functions. If prayers to the Roman gods failed to produce the desired effect, the Romans sometimes introduced foreign deities. In 293 BCE during a pestilence, for example, the Romans consulted the oracular Sibylline books, which directed them to send a mission to Epidaurus to bring the god Asklepios to Rome. Two years later they did so. According to the legend, Asklepios took the form of a serpent and boarded a Roman ship, which carried him to Rome, where he disembarked on Tiber Island. The Romans built a temple for him, and he was worshiped as Aesculapius [3.4].

The Romans also personified forces like fever, which came to be represented as a goddess (Febris) whose anger might be propitiated by remedies for disease. They believed that every natural function was under the protection of a particular deity. Hence every stage of life, including conception, gestation, and birth, came under the protection of a numen, and the favor of the appropriate spirit or deity was sought. Given the dangers of childbearing, which claimed the lives of many women, a Roman matron might appeal to any number of Roman goddesses in childbirth, although through a process of syncretism Juno/Lucina and Diana came to replace most of the others. Incantations and magical formulas were often recited together with the laying on of hands, which was thought to transfer the power of a deity and promote fertility or provide safety in childbearing or healing [3.3].

The first recorded physician to practice medicine in Rome, probably as a public physician, was Archagathus, a Greek who settled in Rome in 219 BCE. Although he was initially well received, he relied heavily on surgery and cautery, which damaged his reputation and gained him the title of *carnifex* (executioner) [3.5]. Many subsequent Greek physicians were attracted to Rome, where they enjoyed great popularity in a city that had never before had professional medical practitioners. Yet some Romans, like Cato the Elder and the encyclopedist of the imperial period, Pliny the Elder (23/24–79 CE), distrusted physicians and relied on popular folk medicine long after the introduction and widespread acceptance of theoretical Greek medicine. Pliny included many folk and magical remedies in his influential *Natural History*, as did the antiquarian Varro in his work *On Agriculture* [3.8].

As Rome conquered the Mediterranean world in the second and first centuries BCE, Roman culture underwent many rapid changes owing to eastern influences and Greek thought. Some Romans abandoned their traditional religion for philosophy or skepticism, whereas others supplemented the mechanical and formal civic religion with eastern religions. The influence of foreign beliefs, such as astrology and magic, spread throughout Italy as soldiers returned from foreign campaigns and slaves were brought to Italy. Although amulets had always been worn to ward off disease and personal disaster, magicians and exorcists soon abounded, selling charms and incantations to exorcise demons or to heal diseases. The belief that certain animals, plants, and precious stones possessed occult properties, which released magical forces through manipulation, influenced healing practices. Astrologers became popular in Rome by the first century CE, and some physicians began to integrate astrology into their medicine [3.20]. Even the distinguished and learned physician Galen [3.10] held that the condition of patients was affected by the course of the moon and the planets.

However, it was the spread of mystery religions that more than any other factor produced new forms of popular religious belief. From Egypt and Asia Minor came many cults that offered a personal satisfaction not found in the formal religion of Rome. They were often modified and westernized by their contact with the Greeks. The most prominent were those of Isis and Sarapis from Egypt, Mithra from Persia, and Magna Mater (Great Mother) from Asia Minor. These cults sometimes offered religious healing, most commonly by means of astrology, magic, divination, or the use of herbs and incantations. Although the cult of Asklepios was introduced into Rome in 291 BCE, it was not until the first century CE that his temple on Tiber Island came to be a popular healing site. By the second century CE Pergamum in Asia Minor had supplanted Epidaurus as the center of healing by Asklepios, and the nature of the cures performed by Asklepios seems to have undergone some modification. To claims of miraculous healing by the god were added therapeutics that were not very different from those that a physician might prescribe. In place of supernatural cures through incubation, Asklepios's priests often recommended practical regimens of exercise, swimming, dietary changes, and purgatives to incubants. We can see this in the detailed accounts of the second-century hypochondriac Aelius Aristides, who was a devotee of Asklepios and a frequent visitor to Pergamum [3.11; cf. 3.12], though there were critics, especially Christians, of temple healing as well [3.13].

Among the eastern influences that became more prominent in the imperial period (30 BCE–476 CE) was belief in the power of demons. In ancient Middle Eastern cultures, such as Mesopotamia and Egypt, demons had been an important part of the religious landscape, and diseases were often attributed to them. In the Greek and Roman cultures, belief in the demonic etiology of disease was generally absent except in cases of pathological conditions that were unexplained, such as epilepsy and insanity, especially after the advent of Greek medicine with its naturalistic understanding of disease. While belief in demons was widespread among the Romans [3.17], few in the Roman imperial period attributed disease to demons. One faith tradition that did was that of the Gnostics, who believed that diseases themselves were demons, which might be expelled by the use of magical formulas [3.19]. Jews who returned to Palestine from Babylon beginning in 538 BCE brought a belief in demons with them, and there are references to the activity of demons and to exorcism in Jewish literature. Both reflect syncretic elements in intertestamental or Second Temple Judaism. This minority view was held by some Jews (see the folk cure for demons in Tobit 6:7). The Jewish sect of the Essenes is known to have practiced exorcism, and Jewish exorcists, such as Eleazar, gained prominence in the wider Roman world [3.16]. There were other celebrated itinerant wonder-workers and healers as well, such as Apollonius of Tyana, who practiced exorcism and attracted much attention [3.18]. Miraculous healing was even attributed to Emperor Vespasian [3.14].

Throughout the history of the Greek and Roman cultures, a medical pluralism generally prevailed. There were always healing cults of various gods and heroes available, including both indigenous and foreign deities. The extent of the belief in magic, astrology, and demonic activity varied over the centuries of classical antiquity, and many who were childless or ill sought the advice of oracles [3.15]. Beginning in the fifth century BCE, natural healing, whether by empirics or by practitioners of theoretical medicine, had become a widely accepted, but not an exclusive, means of healing. Although many physicians considered Asklepios (Aesculapius) their patron, the medicine they practiced was devoid of religious or magical elements. Sources besides medical authors attest—usually indirectly but sometimes directly—to this expectation in classical antiquity. For example, the tragedian Sophocles (496–406 BCE) has one of his characters say, "No good physician (*iatros*) chants incantations over a malady that needs the knife" (*Ajax* 581–82).

Sophocles's view was shared by the jurisconsult Ulpian (d. 228 CE). Ulpian did not deny that alternative healing practices might prove efficacious under some circumstances. But he maintained that those who called themselves physicians were not effective physicians or even physicians at all if they engaged in magical practices. One of the greatest legacies of classical culture is a theoretically based medicine that, irrespective of the enormous changes and developments over the past two and a half millennia, has been the expectation of those in Western cultures who have chosen to consult a physician or surgeon rather than an alternative healer.

## TEXTS

---

### 3.1
### Roman numina
Augustine, *City of God*[1]

*The early Romans were an agricultural and pastoral people. The first phase of Roman religion reflected the outlook of a community of shepherds and farmers who looked for divine protection and blessings for their crops and herds. They were animists who worshiped spirits that they called numina (sing., numen), undefined and indistinct presences that had no human form or moral traits, such as virtues and vices. Some either did not have gender or their sex was unknown. In a well-known passage, Augustine (354–430 CE) described the primitive Roman religion in which there were hundreds of numina.*

But how is it possible to mention in one part of this book all the names of gods or goddesses, which the Romans scarcely could comprise in great volumes, distributing among these divine powers their peculiar functions concerning separate things? They did not even think that the care of their lands should be entrusted to any one god; but they entrusted their farms to the goddess Rumina, and the ridges of the mountains to the god Jugatinus; over the hills they placed the goddess Collatina, over the valleys, Vallonia. Nor could they even find one Segetia so potent that they could commend their cereal crops entirely to her care; but so long as their seed grain was still under the ground, they desired to have the goddess Seia watch over it; then, when it was already above ground and formed standing grain, they set over it the goddess Segetia; and when the grain was collected and stored, they entrusted it to the goddess Tutilina, that it might be kept safe. Who would not have thought the goddess Segetia sufficient to protect the standing grain until it had passed from the first green blades to the dry ears? Yet she was not enough for men who loved a multitude of gods. . . . Therefore they set Proserpina over the germinating seeds; over the joints and knobs of the stems, the god Nodutus; over the sheaths enfolding the ears, the goddess Volutina; when the sheaths opened and the spikes emerged, it was ascribed to the goddess Patelana; when the stems were of the same height as new ears, because the ancients described this equalizing by the term *hostire*, it was ascribed to the goddess Hostilina; when the grain was in flower, it was dedicated to the goddess Flora; when full of milk, to the god Lacturnus; when maturing, to the goddess Matuta; when the crop was "runcated"—that is, removed from the soil—to the goddess Runcina.

## 3.2
## The lectisternium
### Livy, *History of Rome*[2]

*Following an unusually severe winter in which the Tiber River was frozen over and a summer that brought an incurable plague, the Romans assumed that the gods were angry. To determine the reason, the Senate ordered an examination of the Sibylline books, a collection of prophecies of the Cumaean Sibyl that was made for consultation in times of emergency. Accordingly the Senate established the Greek rite of lectisternium, in which the gods were treated at public expense as if they were guests at a banquet. A festival of eight days was proclaimed, during which wooden statues of three pairs of gods (Apollo and Latona, Diana and Hercules, Mercury and Neptune) were placed in reclining positions on couches that were covered with rich robes, and a banquet was prepared for them. Not only did this ritual end the plague, but it also became a celebration in which everyone in the city enjoyed a banquet and general festivities and doubtless relieved the pent-up frustration from the natural disasters that the Romans had experienced.*

The severe winter was succeeded, whether in consequence of the sudden change from such inclement weather to the opposite extreme, or for some other reason, by a summer that was noxious and baleful to all living creatures. Unable to discover what caused the incurable ravages of this distemper, or would put an end to them, the senate voted to consult the Sibylline Books. The duumvirs in charge of the sacred rites then celebrated the first lectisternium ever held in Rome, and for the space of eight days sacrificed to Apollo, to Latona and Diana, to Hercules, to Mercury and to Neptune, spreading three couches for them with all the splendour then attainable. They also observed the rite in their homes. All through the city, they say, doors stood wide open, all kinds of viands were set out for general consumption, all comers were welcomed, whether known or not, and men even exchanged kind and courteous words with personal enemies; there was a truce to quarreling and litigation; even prisoners were loosed from their chains for those days, and they scrupled thenceforth to imprison men whom the gods had thus befriended.

## 3.3
## The festival of Lupercalia
Plutarch, *Life of Romulus*[3]

*The Lupercalia was a Roman festival that was celebrated on February 15. It began with the sacrifice of a goat and a dog at the Lupercal, a cave below the Palatine Hill, in honor of the god Faunus. Youths wearing girdles made from the skins of animals that had been sacrificed ran around the Palatine Hill striking anyone they met, especially women, with strips of goatskin. This ritual beating combined rites of purification with fertility magic and was supposed to increase the ability of the women who had received the lashings to conceive and bear children.*

The Lupercalia, judging from the time of its celebration, would seem to be a feast of purification, for it is observed on the *dies nefasti* of the month of February, which one may interpret to signify *purification*, and the very day of the feast was in ancient days called *Febrata*; but the name of the holiday has the meaning of the Greek Lycaea, and it seems thus to be of great antiquity. . . . And we see the Luperci begin their course from the place where they say Romulus was exposed. But the actual ceremonies make the reason for the name hard to surmise; for there are goats killed; then two youths of noble birth are brought to the priests, some of whom touch their foreheads with a bloody knife, while others at once wipe it off with wool dipped in milk. The youths must laugh after their foreheads are wiped. Next, having cut the goats' skins into strips, the youths run about naked, except for something about their middle, lashing all they meet with the thongs; and the young wives do not avoid their blows, fancying that they will thus promote conception and easy childbirth.

## 3.4
## The introduction of Asklepios into Rome
Anonymous, *On Famous Men*[4]

*After a plague broke out in Rome in 293 BCE, the Romans sent an official dele-*
*gation to Greece to bring the god Asklepios to Rome from his temple in Epidaurus.*
*A sacred serpent, the incarnation of Asklepios, boarded the ship. The serpent*
*departed of its own accord to Tiber Island from the dock in Rome on January 1,*
*291 BCE. Tiber Island thereafter became a healing center, where the god was*
*worshiped as Aesculapius. Any sick slave who was abandoned there would,*
*upon being healed, receive his or her freedom.*

The Romans on account of a pestilence, at the instructions of the Sibylline
books, sent ten envoys under the leadership of Quintus Ogulnius to bring
Aesculapius from Epidaurus. When they had arrived there and were mar-
veling at the huge statue of the god, a serpent glided from the temple, an
object of veneration rather than of horror, and to the astonishment of all
made its way through the midst of the city to the Roman ship, and curled
itself up in the tent of Ogulnius. The envoys sailed to Antium, carrying the
god, where through the calm sea the serpent made its way to a nearby temple
of Aesculapius, and after a few days returned to the ship. And when the ship
was sailing up the Tiber, the serpent leaped on the nearby island, where a
temple was established to him. The pestilence subsided with astonishing
speed.

## 3.5
## Greek physicians in Rome
Pliny, *Natural History*[5]

*The early Romans, like the Israelites before they were influenced by Greek cul-*
*ture, had no native tradition of professional physicians. In 219 BCE a Greek*
*physician by the name of Archagathus was invited to Rome and given Roman*
*citizenship as well as a space in which to practice. It is unlikely that he was the*
*first physician in Rome but he may have been the first public physician, paid a*
*salary by the state to ensure that Romans would have at least minimal pro-*
*fessional medical attention. The Romans were not used to his rough methods*
*of surgery, however, and reacted against them. But as the Romans grew used to*
*the treatment that physicians could offer, the practice of granting citizenship*

*to Greek physicians to encourage them to settle in Rome became customary. Both Julius Caesar and Emperor Augustus granted citizenship to immigrant physicians, nearly all of whom were Greek.*

Cassius Hemina, one of our most ancient writers, is authority for the statement that the first physician that came to Rome was Archagathus, the son of Lysanias, who came over from the Peloponnesus in the 535th year of the city, in the consulship of Lucius Aemilius and Marcus Livius. He states also that the Roman citizenship was granted him, and that he had a shop provided for his practice at the public expense at the Acilian Crossway; that he was a remarkable healer of wounds; that at the beginning his arrival was extraordinarily welcome, but that soon afterwards, from his cruelty in cutting and cauterizing, he acquired the name of *Carnifex* [executioner], and brought his art and physicians into disrepute.

This may be most clearly understood from the words of Marcus Cato, whose authority does not need to be bolstered by his triumph and censorship—so high does it rank of itself. I shall, therefore, cite his own words:

"Concerning those Greeks, son Marcus, I will speak to you in the proper place. I will show you the results of my own experience at Athens: that it is a good idea to dip into their literature but not to learn it thoroughly. I shall convince you that they are a most iniquitous and intractable people, and you may take my word as the word of a prophet: whenever that nation shall bestow its literature upon us, it will corrupt everything, and all the sooner if it sends its physicians here. They have conspired among themselves to murder all foreigners with their medicine, a profession which they exercise for money in order that they may win our confidence and dispatch us all the more easily. They also commonly call us barbarians, and stigmatize us more foully than other peoples, by giving us the appellation of Opici [philistines]. I forbid you to have anything to do with physicians."

### 3.6

### Cato the Elder

Plutarch, *Life of Cato the Elder*[6]

*Marcus Cato the Elder (234–149 BCE) was born of peasant stock. His legal and rhetorical abilities gained the attention of several members of the Roman ruling elite, especially L. Valerius Flaccus, who introduced him to public life. As a* novus homo, *or talented "new man," in Roman politics, he became one of the greatest orators of his day and rose quickly to hold high office in Rome, including the consulship in 195 BCE and the censorship in 184 BCE. He became celebrated for his conservatism in moral, social, and economic matters. His pride in traditional Roman values led to his distrust of everything Greek, whose influence he saw becoming especially prominent in such prominent fields as philosophy and medicine. He denounced Greek physicians in a letter to his son Marcus (Cato the Younger).*

However, Cato's dislike of the Greeks was not confined to philosophers: he was also deeply suspicious of the Greek physicians who practised in Rome. He had heard of Hippocrates's celebrated reply, when he was called upon to attend the king of Persia for a fee amounting to many talents, and declared that he would never give his services to barbarians who were enemies of Greece. Cato maintained that all Greek physicians had taken an oath of this kind, and urged his son not to trust any of them. He himself had compiled a book of recipes and used them for the diet or treatment of any members of his household who fell ill. He never made his patients fast, but allowed them to eat herbs and morsels of duck, pigeon, or hare. He maintained that this diet was light and thoroughly suitable for sick people, apart from the fact that it often produced nightmares, and he claimed that by following it he kept both himself and his family in perfect health.

### 3.7
### A Roman incantation
Cato the Elder, *On Agriculture*[7]

*The introduction of Greek medicine into Rome, in spite of its popularity, did not wholly replace traditional Roman folk medicine, in which magical incantations played an important part. Romans employed magical formulas, sounds, tunes, and invocation of the name of a god or a demon for healing. Sometimes these were uttered or chanted to accompany charms or various concoctions. Many of these practices remained unchanged over the centuries and were incorporated into collections of medical folklore that were included in books on agriculture, such as those of Cato and Varro. In the tradition of the Roman paterfamilias, Cato used incantations and popular remedies in administering folk medicine to members of his family and to his slaves. Here he employs an incantation, with*

*Latin gibberish, along with sympathetic magic. He included it in his treatise on agriculture (de Agricultura), which became a classic work on administering a large estate. Romans continued for centuries to use incantations in place of Greek medicine or, likely more often, to supplement it.*

If something is out of joint, it can be set by the following spell: Take a green reed, four or five feet long, split it in the middle, and let two men hold it to their hips. Begin to recite the following formula: *moetas vaeta daries dardaries abstataries dissunapiter*, until the parts come together. Put iron on top of it. When the two parts have come together and touch each other, grip them with your hand, make a cut left and right, tie it onto the dislocation or the fracture, and it will heal. But you must recite every day *huat huat huat ista sistas sistardannabou dannastra*.

### 3.8
### A traditional incantation
Varro, *On Agriculture*[8]

*M. Terentius Varro (116–27 BCE) was a philologist and antiquarian who is credited with editing 490 books. Among the best known was* Rerum rusticarum, *book 3,* On Agriculture, *by which he hoped to encourage a new interest in farming. In it he preserved many quotations from older writers. In this incantation, the feet that touch the earth are believed to transmit their pain to it. Folk healers often used spittle and recommended a regimen of fasting or a change in diet to promote healing.*

I have heard Tarquenna say that when a man's feet begin hurting he can cure them by thinking of you. [Therefore say:] "I remember you; heal my feet. Let the earth take hold of my illness; let soundness remain in my feet." One should recite this three times nine times, touching the earth, and spitting on it. Do it while fasting.

### 3.9
### An incantation
Marcellus Empiricus, *On Remedies*[9]

*Marcellus of Bordeaux was a Christian physician, perhaps of the fifth century CE, whose* de Medicamentis (On Remedies) *was a mixture of pharmacology, herbal lore, folk medicine, and spells. The spell here includes a magical gesture to accompany the incantation. Although the incantations of Cato, Varro, and Marcellus are separated by several centuries, the magic is much the same. Instructions like these were passed from generation to generation because they were thought to be efficacious and therefore enjoyed wide appeal, like folk remedies everywhere.*

Be fasting [or sober] when you recite [the following]. Touch the affected part of the body with three fingers, the thumb, the middle, and the ring finger, with the other two extended outwards. Then say: "Go away, whether begun today or begun earlier, whether created today or created earlier. This sickness, this disease, this pain, this swelling, this redness, this goiter, this tonsil [growth?], this abscess, this inflammation [swelling], this [infected] gland, and these little [infected] glands I call out, I take out, I declare out [and gone] by this magic, from these limbs and bones."

## 3.10
## Galen's teleology
### Galen, *On the Usefulness of the Parts of the Body*[10]

*Galen was born and raised in Pergamum, a wealthy and important city in western Asia Minor, in 129 CE. In 161, at the age of thirty-three, he left Pergamum for Rome, where he quickly established a reputation as a successful physician and made many prominent acquaintances. He gained the attention of Emperor Marcus Aurelius (r. 161–180 CE) and was a court physician from 169 until his death around 216 CE. His position gave him the leisure to pursue medical research, writing, and lecturing, which he did with great success for a half century.*

*Galen's writings reveal a strong teleological emphasis. He believed that everything was made by the Creator (Plato's Demiurge) for a divine purpose and that the entire creation bore witness to his benevolence. In his treatise* On the Usefulness of the Parts of the Body, *written around 170 CE, he expressed the belief that true piety lies in recognizing and explaining the wisdom, power, and excellence of the creation rather than in offering a multitude of sacrifices. He accepted the Aristotelian principle that nature does nothing in vain, and he attempted to show that every organ was designed to serve a particular function. In its minutest details the human body exhibits its divine origin. Galen's teleological emphasis explains why his otherwise naturalistic but pagan pathology and therapeutics transitioned so well into Christian and modern practice.*

It is time now for you, my reader, to consider which chorus you will join, the one that gathers around Plato, Hippocrates, and the others who admire the works of Nature, or the one made up of those who blame her because she has not arranged to have the superfluities discharged through the feet. . . . But if I should speak further of such fatted cattle, right-thinking men would justly censure me and say that I was desecrating the sacred discourse which I am composing as a true hymn of praise to our Creator. And I consider that I am really showing him reverence not when I offer him unnumbered hecatombs of bulls and burn incense of cassia worth ten thousand talents, but when I myself first learn to know his wisdom, power, and goodness, and then make them known to others. I regard it as proof of perfect goodness that one should will to order everything in the best possible way, not grudging benefits to any creature, and therefore we must praise him as good. But to have discovered how everything should best be ordered is the height of wisdom, and to have accomplished his will in all things is proof of his invincible power.

Then do not wonder so greatly at the beautiful arrangement of the sun, moon, and the whole chorus of stars, and do not be so struck with amazement at the size of them, their beauty, ceaseless motion, and ordered revolutions that things here on earth will seem trivial and disorganized in comparison; for here too you will find displayed the same wisdom, power, and foresight. Consider well the material of which a thing is made, and cherish no idle hope that you could put together from the catamenia [menses] and semen an animal that would be deathless, exempt from pain, endowed with never-ending motion, and as radiantly beautiful as the sun. You should rather estimate the art of the creator of all things just as you judge the art of Phidias. Now perhaps you are struck with admiration of the decoration covering the image of Zeus at Olympia, its gleaming ivory, its massive gold, and great size of the whole statue, and if you saw such a statue made of clay, you would perhaps turn away in contempt. Not so, however, the man who is an artist and able to recognize the art employed in the work; no, he commends Phidias equally, even if he sees him working in cheap wood, common stone, wax, or clay. For the uncultivated man sees beauty in material, whereas it is the art itself that seems beautiful to the artist. Come, then, let us make you skillful in Nature's art so that we may call you no longer an uncultivated person, but a natural philosopher instead. Disregard differences of material and look only at the naked art itself, keeping in mind when you inspect the structure of the eye and the foot that the one is an instrument of vision and the other of locomotion. If you think it proper for the eyes to be made of material like the sun's or for the feet to be pure gold instead of bones and skin, you are forgetting the substance of which you have been formed. . . .

Who will deny that the foot is a small, ignoble part of an animal? And we know full well that the sun is grand and the most beautiful thing in the whole universe. But observe where in the whole universe was the proper place for the sun, and where in the animal the foot had to be placed. In the universe the sun had to be set in the midst of the planets, and in the animal the foot must occupy the lowest position. How can we be sure of this? By assuming a different location for them and seeing what would follow. If you put the sun lower down where the moon is now, everything here would be consumed by fire, and if you put it higher, near Pyroeis or Phaethon, no part of the earth would be habitable because of the cold. The size and character of the sun are qualities inherent in its nature, but its particular position in the universe is the work of One who has arranged it so. For you could find no better place in the whole universe for a body of the size and character of the sun, and in the body of an animal you could find no better place for the foot than the one it occupies. You should observe that the same skill has been employed in locating both sun and foot. (I am intentionally comparing the noblest of the stars with the lowliest member of the animal body.) What is more insignificant than the heel? Nothing. But it could not be better located in any other place. What is nobler than the sun? Nothing. But neither could the sun be better located anywhere else in the whole universe.

What is the grandest and most beautiful of created things? The universe, as everyone admits. But the Ancients, well-versed in Nature, say that an animal is, so to speak, a little universe, and you will find the same wisdom displayed by the Creator in both his works. Then show me, you say, a sun in the body of an animal. What a thing to ask! Are you willing to have the sun formed from the substance of blood, so prone to putrefy and so filthy? Wretched fellow, you are mad! This, and not failure to make offerings and burn incense, is true sacrilege. I will not, indeed, show you the sun in the body of an animal, but I will show you the eye, a very brilliant instrument, resembling the sun as closely as is possible [for a part located] in the body of an animal. I will explain the position of the eye, its size, shape, and all its other qualities, and I will show that everything about it is so beautifully ordered that it could not possibly be improved.

## 3.11
## Aelius Aristides and Asklepios

*Aelius Aristides (117/129–189 CE) was a well-born Greek sophist (a teacher and professional lecturer). A celebrated speaker, he traveled throughout the Roman Empire giving lectures and orations before distinguished audiences, including the emperor. At the age of twenty-six he began to suffer a variety of illnesses, many of which we today would call psychosomatic, which made him an invalid for twelve years. He sought the aid of Asklepios, of whom he became a lifelong devotee and who (Aristides believed) spoke to him and healed him through visions, dreams, and oracles, most often at the temple at Pergamum. Aristides frequently contrasted the advice given by physicians with that of Asklepios, who was always right while the physicians were often wrong. In his* Sacred Tales, *Aelius Aristides recorded his illnesses and the extraordinary cures that the god provided. The following is a sample of his symptoms and the therapies that Asklepios or his priests ordered.*

Aelius Aristides, *Sacred Tales*[11]

And a tumor grew from no apparent cause, at first as it might be for anyone else, and next it increased to an extraordinary size, and my groin was distended, and everything was swollen and terrible pains ensued, and a fever for some days. At this point, the doctors cried out all sorts of things, some said surgery, some said cauterization by drug, or that an infection would arise and I must surely die. But the god gave a contrary opinion and told me to endure and foster the growth. And clearly there was no choice between listening to the doctors or to the god. But the growth increased even more, and there was much dismay. Some of my friends marveled at my endurance, others criticized me because I acted too much on account of dreams, and some even blamed me for being cowardly, since I neither permitted surgery nor again suffered any cauterizing drugs. But the god remained firm throughout and ordered me to bear up with the present circumstances. He said that this was wholly for my safety, for the source of this discharge was located above, and these gardeners did not know where they ought to turn the channels.

Then we were ordered to do many strange things. Of what I remember, there was a race, which it was necessary to run unshod in winter time. And again horseback riding, a most difficult matter. And I also remember some such thing. When the harbor was stormy from a southwest wind and the boats being tossed about, I had to sail across to the opposite side, and having eaten honey and acorns, to vomit, and so the purge was complete. All these things were done while the inflamed tumor was at its worst and was spreading right up to my navel. Finally the Saviour indicated on the same night the same thing to me and to my foster father—for Zosimus was then alive—, so that I sent to him to tell him what the god had said, but he himself came to see me to tell me what he had heard from the god. There was a certain drug, whose particulars I do not remember, except that it contained salt. When we applied this, most of the growth quickly disappeared, and at dawn my friends were present, happy and incredulous. From here on, the doctors stopped their criticisms, expressed extraordinary admiration for the providence of the god in each particular, and said that it was some other greater disease, which he secretly cured. They considered in what way the loose skin (left from the tumor) would arrange itself. Now it seemed to them that there was full need of surgery, for it would not otherwise go back to normal. And they thought it right that I grant this, for now the God's part had been done. He did not even allow them this. But there was a remarkably great lesion and all my skin seemed to change. And he commanded me to smear on an egg and so cured me. And he brought everything back together, so that after a few days had passed, no one was able to find on which thigh the tumor had been, but they were both unscarred in every respect.

Aelius Aristides, *Sacred Tales*[12]

*The usual medical procedure at the temples of Asklepios was incubation. A pilgrim would sleep in the abaton (sanctuary) overnight. During the night the god would appear to him in a dream or a vision. In this narrative Aelius Aristides described the overpowering feeling that he experienced in the presence of Asklepios. After awakening the next morning, he spoke to a minister (sacristan), who told him that his colleague had dreamed the same dream that Aristides had, which confirmed to him that the god had indeed come to him. As a result of the vision Aristides obtained relief from his symptoms. Divine healing provided comfort and an assurance of the god's compassion that natural medicine could not offer, and, as a kind of placebo effect, incubation was likely a powerful component in the healing process.*

The other temple warden was Philadelphus. On the same night this man had a dream vision which I too had, but somehow a little different. Philadelphus dreamed—for so much can I remember—that there was a multitude of men in the Sacred Theater, who wore white garments and were assembled because of the God, and that standing among them, I spoke and hymned the God, and that I said many different things, and how many another time he averted my fate and recently when he found the wormwood and commanded me to drink it diluted with vinegar, so that I might not be nauseated. And he reported a certain sacred ladder, I believe, and the presence and certain wonderful powers of the God. Philadelphus dreamed these things. But the following happened to me. I dreamed that I stood at the propylaea of the Temple. And many others were also gathered together, as whenever there is a purificatory ceremony. And they wore white garments, and the rest was of an appropriate form. Here I cried out other things to the God and called him "the arbiter of fate," since he assigned men their fates. And my words began with my own circumstances. And after this there was wormwood, made clear in some way. It was made clear as possible, just as countless other things clearly contained the presence of the God. For there was a seeming, as it were, to touch him and to perceive that he himself had come, and to be between sleep and waking, and to wish to look up and to be in anguish that he might depart too soon, and to strain the ears and to hear some things as in a dream, some as in a waking state. Hair stood straight, and there were tears with joy, and the pride of the heart was inoffensive. And what man could describe these things in words? If any man has been initiated, he knows and understands. After these things had been seen, when it was dawn, I summoned the doctor Theodotus. And when he came, I recounted my dreams to him. He marvelled at how divine they were, and was at a loss as to what he should do, since he feared the excessive weakness of my body in winter time. For I lay indoors during many successive months. Therefore we thought that it was no worse to send also for the temple warden Asclepiacus. At that time I was living in his house, and besides I was accustomed to share many of my dreams with him. The temple warden came. And we did not get the chance to begin the conversation, but he began to report to us. "Just now," he said, "I have come from my partner"—meaning Philadelphus. "He himself summoned me. For he saw at night a marvelous vision, important to you." And thus Asclepiacus recounted what Philadelphus saw. When he was summoned by us, Philadelphus himself recounted it again. Since the dreams agreed, now we used the curative, and I drank as much as no one before, and again on the next day as the God gave the same signs. Why should one describe the ease in drinking it, or how much it helped? Therefore to return to my argument,—for as it were he arranged my fate as well—many other oracles before and afterwards were revealed with such help in both ways by similar dreams.

Aelius Aristides, *Sacred Tales*[13]

*The following passage is the best-known regimen ordered by Asklepios that Aelius Aristides recorded in the* Sacred Tales. *It was midwinter, and the god commanded him to smear his body with mud and run around the temple three times before bathing himself in the sacred spring. The north wind was so penetrating that his two companions were overcome with the cold, and one nearly died. On another cold day the god ordered Aristides to cover himself with mud, sit in a courtyard, and call on Zeus for healing. Aristides followed these commands of the god because he saw the actions as providing miracles to relieve his illnesses. The severity of the cures may reflect the frustration of Asklepios's priests at the never-ending complaints of a famous hypochondriac.*

Come let us again recall his commands. It was the vernal equinox, when they daub themselves with mud in honor of the God, and it was impossible for me, if he should not give a sign, to stir myself. Therefore I hesitated. The day, as I remember, was also thoroughly warm. Not many days later, there arose a storm and the north wind stirred up all the heaven, and many black clouds gathered together, and again anew winter weather. In these circumstances, he commanded me to use the mud by the Sacred Well and to bathe there. Therefore even then I afforded a spectacle. So great was the coldness of the mud and air, that I regarded myself lucky to run up to the Well. And the water sufficed me, instead of other warmth. And these things are the first part of the miracle.

On the following night, he commanded me again to use the mud in the same way, and to run in a circle about the Temple three times. And the strength of the north wind was indescribable, and the icy cold increased.

Thus you would not find thick clothing to be suitable covering, but the wind passed through and fell on the ribs like a spear. Therefore some of my comrades, as if wishing to console me, although I did not want this, decided to face the danger and imitate me. I smeared myself with mud and ran around, and permitted the north wind to card me well and fair, and finally going to the Well, I bathed. Of them, one immediately turned back, one was seized with convulsions, and having been taken quickly to a bathhouse, was warmed with much difficulty. But after this, we felt the day as spring.

Again in winter time, with ice and the coldest wind, he ordered me to take some mud, pour it on myself, and sit in the courtyard of the Sacred Gymnasium, calling on Zeus, the highest and best God. This also happened before many spectators.

## 3.12
## The testimony of M. Julius Apellas
### Emma J. Edelstein and Ludwig Edelstein, *Asclepius*[14]

*The temple of Asklepios in Pergamum in Asia Minor flourished in the second century CE, when pilgrims came from throughout the Roman Empire for healing. Marcus Julius Apellas, a Roman, made a journey at the command of Asklepios, whom he had consulted earlier, apparently at another shrine. Apellas experienced a variety of seemingly unrelated symptoms that may have been psychosomatic. In a dream he was told to follow a particular regimen, not dissimilar in some respects to what any physician might prescribe, but it was augmented with the healing touch of the god, which added a supernatural or mystical element. His testimonial was recorded in an inscription, which Asklepios had commanded him to write.*

### In the priesthood of Poplius Aelius Antiochus

I, Marcus Julius Apellas, an Idrian from Mylasa, was sent for by the god, for I was often falling into sickness and was suffering from dyspepsia. In the course of my journey, in Aegina, the god told me not to be so irritable. When I arrived at the temple, he told me for two days to keep my head covered, and for these two days it rained; to eat cheese and bread, celery with lettuce, to wash myself without help, to practice running, to take lemon peels, to soak them in water, near the (spot of the) *akoai* in the bath to press against the wall, to take a walk in the upper portico, to take some passive exercise, to sprinkle myself with sand, to walk around barefoot, in the bathroom, before plunging into the hot water, to pour wine over myself, to bathe without help and to give an Attic drachma to the bath attendant, in common to offer sacrifice to Asclepius, Epione and the Eleusinian goddesses, to take milk with honey. When one day I had drunk milk alone he said, "Put honey in the milk so that it can get through." When I asked of the god to relieve me more quickly I thought I walked out of the abaton near the (spot of the) *akoai* being anointed all over with mustard and salt, while a small boy was leading me holding a smoking censer, and the priest said: "You are cured but you must pay up the thank-offerings." And I did what I had seen, and when I anointed myself with the salts and the moistened mustard I felt pains, but when I bathed I had no pain. That happened within nine days after I had come. He touched my right hand and also my breast. The following day as I was offering sacrifice the flame leapt up and scorched my hand, so that blisters appeared. Yet after a little the hand got well. As I stayed on he said I should use dill along with olive oil against my headaches. I usually did not suffer from headaches. But it happened that after I had studied, my head was congested. After I used the olive oil I got rid of the headache. To gargle with a cold gargle for the uvula—since about that too I had consulted the god—and the same also for the tonsils. He bade me also inscribe this. Full of gratitude I departed well.

## 3.13
### A Christian critique of temple healing
Eusebius, *The Preparation of the Gospel*[15]

*Magic, the art of using preternatural forces to control and manipulate the course of nature, was ubiquitous in the ancient world. Christians condemned magic as the work of demons, while often finding it necessary to tolerate the magical charms and amulets that continued to be used by many converts from paganism. The church historian Eusebius (c. 260–340 CE) rejected all forms of pagan magic, and he offered rational explanations for prophecies that were allegedly given by the gods. He critiqued fraudulent priests, who were "clever men," for expressing oracles in an ambiguous and deceptive way. Without mentioning the god's name, Eusebius claimed that the miraculous healings of Asklepios were caused by hallucinatory or sleep-inducing drugs and aided by priests who solicited information that was used in making prophecies. Additional causes were the fact that healing took place under cover of darkness, and the influence of what today we would term psychosomatic factors, such as the mood of expectation that pilgrims who sought healing brought with them, or their fear of or trust in the god who was part of their religious heritage.*

Even for the pagans it is obvious that lifeless statues are not gods. . . . But let us [now] consider this question: How should one look at the powers lurking in statues? Can one have a pleasant relationship with them? Are they good and truly divine or the very opposite of all this?

If someone were to study this subject thoroughly, he might possibly come to the conclusion that everything is a mystification produced by sorcerers and consists of fraud. Thus would he demolish their [the sorcerers'] prestige by showing that the stories told about them are certainly not the work of a god, and not even the work of an evil daemon. For the oracles in verse, skillfully arranged, are the work of clever men; they are fiction and designed to deceive; they are expressed in such a vague, ambiguous manner as to fit both of two possible outcomes of a prediction quite well.

One might also say that portents which seem miraculous and deceive the masses can be explained by natural causes. For in all of nature there are many kinds of roots, herbs, plants, fruits, stones, as well as the various forces inherent in matter, whether they are dry or humid. Some of them have the power of repelling and driving away; others are magnetic and attract; some can separate and split up, others can assemble and concentrate; others can relax, make wet, rarefy; some save and others destroy; some transform and bring about change in the present condition, one way or another, for a short while or a long time; their effect may be felt by many people or only by a few; some of them lead the way, and others follow; some agree with others and increase and decrease along with them; some are conducive to health and belong in the realm of medical science, while others produce illness and are harmful. Thus certain phenomena are due to the necessary effect of natural causes, and they wax and wane with the moon.

There are thousands of antipathies between living beings, roots and plants: certain perfumes go to the head and make you sleepy, while others produce visions. Moreover, the places, the locations where something is going on, also contribute a great deal, not to mention the instruments and the apparatus which sorcerers have held ready long beforehand to help them in their art. They also benefit from all sorts of outside assistance to bring off their deceit: helpers who receive the visitors with a great show of interest and find out what their business is and what they wish to know. The inner sanctum and the recesses inside the temple, which are not accessible to the public, also hide many secrets. The darkness certainly helps them in their fraudulent scheme, and the mood of expectation, the fear the visitors experience when they think they are approaching the gods, and all the religious prejudices they have inherited from their ancestors.

### 3.14
### Vespasian cures two men
Suetonius, *Life of Vespasian*[16]

*Vespasian was proclaimed emperor by his troops in 69 CE following the short reigns of three generals who had been successively proclaimed emperor after the suicide of Nero. A plebeian and military man, Vespasian lacked the patrician status and reputation usually thought desirable for an aspirant to the throne. In Alexandria he was approached by two men who sought his healing, and he reluctantly responded to their request. (The account is paralleled in Tacitus, Histories 4.81–82 and Dio Cassius 65.8.1–2.) The public event was probably arranged by members of his staff with a view to legitimating his ascendancy to the throne by a display of his thaumaturgic touch, as the "royal touch" did centuries later among French and English kings. By a successful healing, it was thought, Vespasian could gain the reputation of a wonder-worker.*

Vespasian as yet lacked prestige and a certain divinity, so to speak, since he was an unexpected and still new-made Emperor. But these also were given him. A man of the people who was blind, and another who was lame, came to him together as he sat on the tribunal, begging for the help for their disorders which Serapis had promised in a dream. For the god declared that Vespasian would restore the eyes, if he would spit upon them, and give strength to the leg, if he would deign to touch it with his heel. Though he had hardly any faith that this could possibly succeed, and therefore shrank even from making the attempt, he was at last prevailed upon by his friends and tried both things in public before a large crowd; and with success. At this same time, by the direction of certain soothsayers, some vases of antique workmanship were dug up in a consecrated spot at Tegea in Arcadia and among them was an image very like Vespasian.

## 3.15
## The oracle at Dodona
Georg Luck, *Arcana Mundi*[17]

*Dodona was an oracle of Zeus in Epirus, northwest of Greece, to which pilgrims came to consult the god. They wrote questions on lead tablets and submitted them to the priests, who returned answers ostensibly given by Zeus. Many questions, such as the following, were of a personal nature.*

Nicocrateia would like to know to what god she ought to offer sacrifice in order to get well and feel better and make her illness go away.

## 3.16
## Eleazar's exorcism before Vespasian
Josephus, *Jewish Antiquities*[18]

*Belief in demonic possession was brought to Palestine by Jews who returned from the Babylonian captivity after 539 BCE, when the Persian king Cyrus captured Babylon. Exorcism is attested in sources from the Second Temple period of Judaism, beginning with the book of Tobit (third century BCE), which, though fictional, provides the earliest narrative of an exorcism in Hebrew literature. There were several Jewish exorcists and magicians in this period, the most prominent of whom was Eleazar, whose public exorcism of a demon in the presence of Emperor Vespasian (r. 69–79 CE) and his officers and troops was described by the first-century Jewish historian Josephus. In this period Solomon came to be regarded as a celebrated magician and exorcist. He was believed to have composed incantations to cure illnesses and exorcise demons.*

Now so great was the prudence and wisdom which God granted Solomon that he surpassed the ancients, and even the Egyptians, who are said to excel all men in understanding, were not only, when compared with him, a little inferior but proved to fall far short of the king in sagacity. . . . And God granted him knowledge of the art used against demons for the benefit and healing of men. He also composed incantations by which illnesses are relieved, and left behind forms of exorcisms with which those possessed by demons drive them out, never to return. And this kind of cure is of very great power among us to this day, for I have seen a certain Eleazar, a countryman of mine, in the presence of Vespasian, his sons, tribunes and a number of other soldiers, free men possessed by demons, and this was the manner of the cure: he put to the nose of the possessed man a ring which had under its seal one of the roots prescribed by Solomon, and then, as the man smelled it, drew out the demon through his nostrils, and, when the man at once fell down, adjured the demon never to come back into him, speaking Solomon's name and reciting the incantations which he had composed. Then, wishing to convince the bystanders and prove to them that he had this power, Eleazar placed a cup or foot-basin full of water a little way off and commanded the demon, as it went out of the man, to overturn it and make known to the spectators that he had left the man. And when this was done, the understanding and wisdom of Solomon were clearly revealed, on account of which we have been induced to speak of these things, in order that all men may know the greatness of his nature and how God favoured him, and that no one under the sun may be ignorant of the king's surpassing virtue of every kind.

### 3.17
### A pagan theology of demons
Eusebius, *Preparation of the Gospel*[19]

*Beginning in the late second century there was a growing interest in demons among pagans, Christians, and Jews. Demons played an important role in pagan theology, as Eusebius pointed out in the following passage. He identified four main categories of supernatural beings in paganism: a supreme god, the gods, demons (both good and evil), and heroes (humans who had become divine). He argued that pagans, while claiming to worship only the benevolent gods, in fact out of fear worship only the malevolent demons and that demons therefore play a disproportionate role in pagan worship. Christians considered pagan gods to be demons in disguise and viewed all demons as an evil force.*

Those who have a thorough knowledge of pagan theology . . . divide the whole doctrine into four parts: first of all they distinguish the supreme god; they say they know that he rules over everything and that he is the father and the king of all the gods. After him there is a second category of gods; then comes the category of daemons; and as number four they list the heroes. All these, they say, share in the idea of the Good, and thus in a sense lead and in another sense are led, and every substance of this kind, they say, can be called light because it participates in light. But they also say that Evil is in control of what is inferior; this is the category of the evil daemons; there is no friendship between them and the Good; they certainly have an enormous power in the sphere that is totally opposed to the Good; and everything of this kind they call "darkness."

Having distinguished these categories, they say that heaven and the ether as far down as the moon are assigned to the gods; to the daemons, the region around the moon and the atmosphere; to the souls [of the dead], the terrestrial regions and the subterranean spaces. Having established these distinctions, they say that one must first of all worship the gods of heaven and of the ether; then the good daemons; in the third place the souls of the heroes; and in the fourth place one must soothe the evil and malevolent daemons. After they have made these distinctions in theory, they confuse everything in practice, and instead of worshiping all the powers mentioned, they worship only the evil powers and serve them exclusively, as I will show in a later part of my discussion.

## 3.18
## An exorcism by Apollonius of Tyana
### Philostratus, *Life of Apollonius of Tyana*[20]

*Apollonius of Tyana was born in Cappadocia, and his life spanned most of the first century CE. He was a wonder-worker of a kind that was characteristic of the early Roman Empire. A wandering ascetic philosopher who visited India, he practiced exorcism and miraculous healing and claimed the gift of clairvoyance, allegedly foreseeing the deaths of the emperors Nero and Domitian. Apollonius was the subject of a fictionalized biography by Philostratus that was commissioned by Empress Julia Domna, from which the following account of an exorcism is taken.*

The discussion was interrupted when among the wise men a messenger appeared. He brought with him some Indians who needed help. Among others, he presented a poor woman who implored them to do something for her son. She said that he was sixteen years old and had been possessed by a daemon for two years, and that the daemon had a sarcastic and deceitful nature.

When one of the wise men asked her on what basis she made this claim, she answered: "My son is rather good-looking, and the daemon is in love with him and won't allow him to be normal, or go to school or to archery practice, or to stay at home, but drives him out to desert places. The boy does not even have his own voice, but speaks in a deep, hollow tone, the way grown-up men do, and when he looks at me, his eyes don't seem to be his own. All this makes me cry and scratch my cheeks. I try to talk sense into him, to a certain degree, but he doesn't even know me. As I was planning to come to you—in fact I have been planning it since last year—the daemon made himself known to me, using my son as a mouthpiece, and told me that he was the ghost of a man who had been killed in a war a long time ago, and he had been very much in love with his wife at the time he was killed. But he had been dead for only three days when his wife married another man, thus mocking her previous marriage. Since then (the daemon said) he had begun to loath the love of women and had transferred himself into this boy. He promised to give the boy many precious and useful gifts if I would not denounce him to you. This made an impression on me, but he has put me off again and again; he has complete control over my house, and his intentions are neither reasonable nor honorable."

Apollonius asked . . . if the boy was nearby. She said "No"; she had tried very hard to make him come here, "but the daemon," she said, "threatens to throw me into a crevice or {off} a precipice and to kill my son if I bring him here for trial." "Be of good cheer," the wise man said, "for he will not kill him when he reads this," and he snatched a letter from his neckpiece and gave it to her. The letter, of course, was addressed to the daemon and contained the most appalling threats.

### 3.19
### The Gnostic belief that demons cause illness
Plotinus, *Enneads*[21]

*Unlike the Babylonians and Egyptians, most people in the classical world, including Christians, did not attribute disease to demons. The faith communities that did were the Gnostics and some sectarian Jewish groups, such as the Essenes. Gnostics formed a variety of sects that claimed to have a secret knowledge (gnosis) that was denied to ordinary people. They employed esoteric forms of this knowledge, according to Plotinus, that included magic, by which they claimed to be able to control natural forces and to exorcise demons. Plotinus (205–269/70 CE) was a distinguished Neoplatonist philosopher who, while believing in magic, rejected Gnostic esoteric beliefs and argued that disease is better explained by natural causes than by magic.*

There is another way in which they [the Gnostics] grossly insult the purity of the higher powers. When they write out incantations, as if they were addressing those powers—not only the soul, but the powers above as well—what else are they doing but, if I may say so, forcing [the gods] to obey magic, to be led by witchcraft, charms, and formulas spoken by them? [Does this mean that] any of us who is highly accomplished in the art of reciting such formulas in the right way—songs and sounds, breathing and hissing—and everything else which works, according to their writings, has control over the higher powers?

If they are reluctant to put it this way, [let me ask,] how can incorporeal things be affected by sound? By the kind of phrases they use to make their theories look more sublime, they take away, without realizing it, the sublimity of those powers. They claim that they can cure themselves of diseases; if they mean that they can do this by self-discipline and a rational way of life, "fine," as the philosophers would put it. But in fact they assume that diseases are caused by daemons, and they claim that they can exorcise the daemons by their words. When they claim this, they may look quite sublime in the eyes of the average person who is in awe of the powers ascribed to magicians, but they would scarcely convince any sensible person [when they assert] that diseases do not have their origin in fatigue, or over-eating, or lack of food, or a process of putrefaction, or, generally speaking, in changes that have their origin inside or outside.

Their treatment of illness makes this clear. If the patient has diarrhea, or if a laxative has been administered, the illness passes through the downward passage and leaves the body. It is the same with bloodletting. Fasting also heals. Does this happen because the daemon has been starving and the drug has made him waste away? Does he sometimes leave at once and sometimes remain inside? If he remains inside, how is it [possible] that the patient is feeling better, even though the daemon is still inside? And if the daemon is there to stay, how is it [possible] that the patient is feeling better, even though the daemon is still inside? Why did he leave—if he actually left? What happened to him? Did he perhaps thrive on the illness? In that case, the illness is different from the daemon. Moreover, if the daemon enters the body without any cause [i.e., in the absence of illness], why are we not always sick? And if there was a cause, why do we need the daemon to get sick? The cause is sufficient to produce a fever. It would be ridiculous to suppose that as soon as the cause operates, the daemon, standing by, moves in at once, as if to reinforce the cause. No, it is quite clear what they mean, what they intend, when they say all this, and for this reason above all—but for other reasons as well—did I mention their doctrine concerning daemons.

## 3.20
## Medical astrology
Ptolemy of Alexandria, *Tetrabiblus*[22]

*Ptolemy of Alexandria (fl. 121–151 CE) was one of the greatest scientific writers of the classical world. His best-known works were the* Almagest *(its Arabic title, by which it became known in the Middle Ages), which summarized all the astronomical knowledge of the time, and his* Geography; *both became the standard handbooks of knowledge in their respective fields for more than a thousand years. Ptolemy also authored the* Tetrabiblus, *excerpted here, which became the most widely used text on technical astrology in European history. In it Ptolemy attempted to provide a scientific explanation of how the heavenly bodies influence the destiny of humans by means of a cosmic sympathy that connects the movements of the planets with the earth. Ptolemy traced the practice of medical astrology to Hellenistic Egypt, where the physician-astrologer would cast a patient's horoscope to gather information regarding the person's health, which would then be used in particularizing medical treatment. Medical astrology was widely practiced in the ancient and medieval worlds, and physicians continued to view it as a helpful tool in prognosis until the eighteenth century.*

As far as [astrological] predictions are concerned, it seems that even if they are not infallible, their potential at least is most impressive. Similarly, prevention works in some cases, even if it does not take care of everything; and even if these cases are few and insignificant, they should be welcomed and appreciated and considered as unusual benefit.

The Egyptians were aware of this. They developed this technique further than anyone else by thoroughly combining medicine with astrological prognosis. They would never have established certain means of prevention or protection or preservation against conditions that exist or are about to exist in the atmosphere, in general or specifically, if they had not been convinced that the future could not be changed or influenced. In fact, they placed the possibility of reacting by a series of natural abilities right after the theory of fate. They combined with the possibility of prediction the useful and beneficial part of the method they called "medical astrology" because they wanted to find out, thanks to astrology, the specific nature of the mixtures in matter and the things that are bound to happen because of the atmosphere and their individual causes. They felt that without this knowledge any remedies must fail, since the same remedies would not be appropriate for all bodies and all affections. On the other hand, their medical knowledge of sympathetic or antipathetic forces in each case and their knowledge of a preventative therapy for an impending illness as well as the cure for an existing disease enabled them as much as possible to prescribe the correct treatment.

## NOTES

1. Augustine, *City of God* 4.8, in Lewis and Reinhold, *Roman Civilization: Sourcebook I*, 130.

2. Livy, *History of Rome* 5.13.4–8, in *Livy, in Fourteen Volumes*.

3. Plutarch, *Life of Romulus* 21.3–5, in Lewis and Reinhold, *Roman Civilization: Sourcebook I*, 480.

4. Anonymous, *On Famous Men* 22.1–3, ibid., 143.

5. Pliny, *Natural History* 29.1.12–14, in W. H. S. Jones, trans., *Natural History*, vol. 8: *Books 28–32* (Cambridge, MA: Harvard University Press, 1963). Loeb Classical Library, vol. 418. Copyright © 1963 by the President and Fellows of Harvard College. Loeb Classical Library is a registered trademark of the President and Fellows of Harvard College.

6. Plutarch, *Life of Cato the Elder* 23 (146).

7. Marcus Cato, *On Agriculture* 160, in Georg Luck, ed. and trans., *Arcana Mundi: Magic and the Occult in the Greek and Roman Worlds: A Collection of Ancient Texts*, 2nd ed. (Baltimore, MD: Johns Hopkins University Press, 2006), 109 (7A). Copyright © 2006 Johns Hopkins University Press. Reprinted with permission of Johns Hopkins University Press.

8. Varro, *On Agriculture* 1.2.27, in Grant, *Ancient Roman Religion*, 38.

9. Marcellus Empiricus, *On Remedies* 15.11, ibid., 38.

10. Galen, *On the Usefulness of the Parts of the Body* 3.1.174–77.

11. Aelius Aristides, *Sacred Tales* 1.62–63, 65–68, in Behr, *Aelius Aristides and the Sacred Tales*.

12. Ibid., 2.30–36.

13. Ibid., 2.74–77.

14. Emma J. Edelstein and Ludwig Edelstein, *Asclepius: A Collection and Interpretation of the Testimonies* (Baltimore, MD: Johns Hopkins University Press, 1998), 1:248. Copyright © 1998 Johns Hopkins University Press. Reprinted with permission of Johns Hopkins University Press.

15. Eusebius, *Preparation of the Gospel* 4.1.6–9, in Luck, *Arcana Mundi* 163–64 (35).

16. Suetonius, *Life of Vespasian* 7, in Suetonius, *Lives of the Caesars*.

17. Wilhelm Dittenberger, *Sylloge Inscriptionum Graecarum*, 3rd ed. (1982), in Luck, *Arcana Mundi* 325 (79, no. 1161).

18. Josephus, *Jewish Antiquities* 8.2.5, in Ralph Marcus, trans., *Jewish Antiquities: Books VII-VIII* (Cambridge, MA: Harvard University Press, first published 1934). Loeb Classical Library, vol. 281. Loeb Classical Library is a registered trademark of the President and Fellows of Harvard College.

19. Eusebius, *Preparation of the Gospel* 4.5.1–3, in Luck, *Arcana Mundi* 276–77 (73).

20. Philostratus, *Life of Apollonius of Tyana* 3.38–39, ibid., 200–201 (50).

21. Plotinus, *Enneads* 2.9.14, ibid., 164–65 (36).

22. Ptolemy of Alexandria, *Tetrabiblus* 1.3.17–19, ibid., 416–17 (117).

# FOUR

# Early Christianity

## INTRODUCTION

The Gospels recount the career of Jesus of Nazareth (c. 4 BCE–c. 30 CE), the founder of Christianity. During a ministry of three years, it is said, Jesus performed more than two dozen instances of miraculous healing, which included restoring to health the blind, the dumb, the deaf, the lame, and lepers [4.1]. The Gospels differentiate between Jesus's miracles and the miracles of conventional exorcists and magicians. While Jesus is said to have cast out demons, the Gospels usually distinguish between his acts of exorcism and of healing (see Matthew 8:16; cf. Mark 6:12 and Acts 19:12). Nor does it appear that either he or his disciples considered demons to be the cause of disease. Several medical conditions are described in the Gospels, including blindness, deafness, fever, paralysis, and dysentery. Most are either ordinary diseases or congenital conditions for which a natural cause is assumed by those who suffer from them. The Gospels differentiate the symptoms of ordinary disease from those that accompany demonic posses-sion, which were usually manifested as erratic or abnormal behavior. Jesus is often said to have healed chronic diseases or congenital conditions for which medical treatment had been unsuccessful (e.g., Mark 5:24–34).

Outside the Gospels and the healings of Jesus there is little reference to miraculous healing in the New Testament. The book of Acts describes a relatively small number of supernatural healings that are attributed to Jesus's disciples (3:1–11, 9:33–34, 14:8–10) [4.4]. They belong to the category of "signs and wonders," which are said to confirm the disciples' apostolic cre-dentials (Acts 14:3). The diseases healed are natural conditions, and none is attributed to demonic etiology. In the New Testament epistles, we do not find any case of sickness that is either healed miraculously or attributed to demonic causation. The epistles suggest that first-century Christians suffered from ordinary illnesses from which they sometimes recovered gradually (e.g., Philippians 2:25–27) and sometimes did not recover (e.g., 2 Timothy 4:20) [4.6]. It does not appear that in the first three centuries of the Christian era supernatural or religious healing played a major role in the church's ministry to the sick.

Leading Christian writers of the early period for the most part exhibited positive views of medicine. Thus Origen (c. 185–c. 254) considered medicine to be "beneficial and essential to mankind" (*Contra Celsum* 3.12) while Tertullian (c. 160–c. 225), who was fond of employing medical analogies in his writings, believed that medicine was appropriate for Christians to use [4.7]. The theme of Jesus as *Christus medicus* (Great Physician) was popular among Christian authors of the second century. But it was used in a metaphorical sense to describe the savior of sin-sick souls, not of physical healing. Medical care, far from being rejected by early Christians, was regarded as a model of the care of the soul.

The early Christian understanding of disease combined theological and medical as well as natural and supernatural elements. Early Christians attributed diseases to one of three sources—God, demons, or nature—but they were not viewed as mutually exclusive. Christians regarded disease as an aspect of the material (rather than the moral) evil that had resulted from the Fall. Within the religious context they had inherited from Judaism, early Christian teaching tended to reject conventional theodicies that viewed suffering as the result of sin [4.2]. Christians looked on illness as the result of natural (if providential) causes, which could be treated by physicians or other healers, of whom a broad spectrum, including midwives, root cutters, herbalists, and folk healers, existed in what has been termed the "medical marketplace" of the classical world. Christians broke bones and contracted diseases like their pagan and Jewish neighbors, for which they ordinarily consulted physicians. When medical or natural means did not avail, they might seek healing by prayer or anointing [4.5]. But in cases for which no relief was possible, Christians were advised to submit patiently to God's will. Early Christian writers repeatedly spoke of suffering as intended by God to produce spiritual maturity (see, e.g., Hebrews 12:7–11; 1 Peter 4:12). Faith and trust in God, they wrote, can transform suffering into a positive experience and nurture Christian graces, such as humility, patience, and dependence on Christ (see, e.g., Romans 5:2–5; James 5:10–11; 2 Corinthians 12:7–10).

From the beginning Christians exhibited a philanthropic spirit in their concern, both personally and corporately, for those in physical need. The model here was Jesus's parable of the good Samaritan [4.3]. This spirit was in marked contrast with that of the classical world, in which there existed little or no religious basis for charity expressed as a personal concern for those who suffered physical distress. Christian concepts of philanthropy were motivated by agape, a self-sacrificing love of one's fellows that bore witness to the love of Christ as reflected in his incarnation and redemptive work on the cross (see, e.g., Matthew 25:35–40; James 1:27). Christians were encouraged to visit the sick privately (Hippolytus, *Apostolic Tradition*, canon 20), while deacons (whose duties largely consisted of the relief of physical want and suffering) were expected to visit the ill (*Apostolic Constitution* 3.19; cf. Polycarp, *Epistle ad Philippians* 6.1).

In the third century, as Christianity grew rapidly in the large cities of the Roman Empire, extensive benevolent work was organized and centered in local congregations. Minor ecclesiastical orders were created to assist deacons in their charitable work. In Rome, for example, the Christian church by 251 had divided the city into seven districts, each the responsibility of a deacon and his assisting clergy. The church supported fifteen hundred widows and others, including the ill, who were suffering and in want (Eusebius, *Ecclesiastical History* 6.43). Adolf Harnack estimated that the Roman church spent between five hundred thousand and one million sesterces each year in support of its charitable ministry.[1] (A sesterce was one-quarter of a denarius, which was a day's wage.) Other churches in the large cities of the empire spent similar sums on charity; the funds were administered by bishops or presbyters.

Beginning in 250 the cities of the Roman Empire experienced a major plague that lasted for fifteen or twenty years and reached epidemic proportions [4.8, 4.9]. When the civic authorities did little to deal with the plague, the Christian churches undertook the systematic care of the victims and the burial of the dead in spite of the fact that Christians were at the time a persecuted minority. There are descriptions of the organization of the care of the sick in Rome, Carthage, and Edessa in Syria [4.10, 4.11]. In Alexandria a medical corps known as the *parabalani* was formed to transport and nurse the sick under the jurisdiction of the patriarch of Alexandria.

The legalization of Christianity by Constantine in 313 resulted in major changes in the church's administration of medical philanthropy. The role of the individual congregation and the laity declined, while that of the bishop, who administered the charitable programs, grew. In the 370s Christians created the first hospital (*xenodochium*), a specifically Christian institution that arose out of the philanthropic ideals of the early church. No similar public organization existed in the classical world. Roman infirmaries (*valetudinaria*) for soldiers and slaves on plantation estates played a much more limited role, and the sick were left to help themselves [4.11].

Hospitals often included an orphanage and houses for the poor and aged in a single complex. Probably the earliest and certainly the most celebrated was the Basileias, founded by Basil the Great, the bishop of Caesarea (in modern Turkey), about 372 CE [4.15]. Hospitals modeled on the Basileias spread quickly in the East and slightly later in the West. The first hospital in the West was founded in Rome about 390 by Fabiola, whose friend Jerome described how she gathered the sick from the public squares of the city, where homeless sick people were often found in the ancient world, and nursed the seriously ill herself (*Epistle* 77.6.1–2) [4.16]. Hospitals were distinctively Christian institutions, and in the fourth century the Roman emperor Julian the Apostate (r. 361–63) sought to emulate the Christians by founding his own system for helping those in need [4.17].

Many of the early Christian hospitals were staffed by monks. Monasticism, which originated in the deserts of Egypt, Palestine, and Syria in the third century, grew out of attempts to deepen the spiritual life among Christians through the renunciation of the world and the practices of self-mortification. The founders of the movement were anchorites or hermits, who sought solitude in the desert, but by the fourth century anchoritic monasticism had in part given way to cenobitic monasticism, in which monks and nuns lived in ordered communities. A strong compassionate impulse in monasticism provided the motivation for monks to serve as lay medical attendants and even as physicians.

The adoption of magical amulets, the growing veneration of relics associated with Christian martyrs, and the new importance that Christian leaders like Augustine and Ambrose placed on miracles of healing signaled a major change in Christian approaches to healing [4.12]. Some of the desert fathers, such as Anthony, the founder of anchoritic monasticism, were credited with miraculous powers to heal the sick [4.13]. At the same time, in a list of miraculous cures that he recorded, Augustine (*City of God* 22.8) assumed a natural etiology for every case [4.12c]. The rapid spread of hospitals at the end of the fourth century suggests that Christians still sought medical assistance for their illnesses, perhaps resorting to supernatural cures when physicians had failed them. And there was a growing emphasis by Christian leaders to show compassion even to the most miserable members of the sick, the lepers [4.14].

## TEXTS

---

### 4.1
### Gospel accounts of Jesus's miracles of healing

*Miracles of healing are assigned a central place in the ministry of Jesus in the Gospels of the New Testament. Some two dozen examples are given of his reported healing of people who were blind, deaf, mute, lame, or otherwise disabled, as well as lepers. Jesus's healings are spoken of as signs of his messianic credentials and as a fulfillment of Old Testament prophecies. But the Gospels make clear that his miracles engendered opposition and hostility from some of the religious leaders of Judaism. Less frequent in the Gospels are accounts of exorcism, which are usually but not invariably distinguished from healing.*

#### a. Jesus heals a crippled woman
Gospel of Luke[2]

[10] Now he was teaching in one of the synagogues on the sabbath. [11] And just then there appeared a woman with a spirit that had crippled her for eighteen years. She was bent over and was quite unable to stand up straight. [12] When Jesus saw her, he called her over and said, "Woman, you are set free from your ailment." [13] When he laid his hands on her, immediately she stood up straight and began praising God. [14] But the leader of the synagogue, indignant because Jesus had cured on the sabbath, kept saying to the crowd, "There are six days on which work ought to be done; come on those days and be cured, and not on the sabbath day." [15] But the Lord answered him and said, "You hypocrites! Does not each of you on the sabbath untie his ox or his donkey from the manger, and lead it away to give it water? [16] And ought not this woman, a daughter of Abraham whom Satan bound for eighteen long years, be set free from this bondage on the sabbath day?"

### b. A girl restored to life and a woman healed
Gospel of Matthew[3]

[18] While he was saying these things to them, suddenly a leader of the synagogue came in and knelt before him, saying, "My daughter has just died; but come and lay your hand on her, and she will live." [19] And Jesus got up and followed him, with his disciples. [20] Then suddenly a woman who had been suffering from hemorrhages for twelve years came up behind him and touched the fringe of his cloak, [21] for she said to herself, "If I only touch his cloak, I will be made well." [22] Jesus turned, and seeing her he said, "Take heart, daughter; your faith has made you well." And instantly the woman was made well. [23] When Jesus came to the leader's house and saw the flute players and the crowd making a commotion, [24] he said, "Go away; for the girl is not dead but sleeping." And they laughed at him. [25] But when the crowd had been put outside, he went in and took her by the hand, and the girl got up. [26] And the report of this spread throughout that district.

### c. Jesus heals two blind men
Gospel of Matthew[4]

[27] As Jesus went on from there, two blind men followed him, crying loudly, "Have mercy on us, Son of David!" [28] When he entered the house, the blind men came to him; and Jesus said to them, "Do you believe that I am able to do this?" They said to him, "Yes, Lord." [29] Then he touched their eyes and said, "According to your faith let it be done to you." [30] And their eyes were opened. Then Jesus sternly ordered them, "See that no one knows of this." [31] But they went away and spread the news about him throughout that district.

### d. Jesus heals one who is mute
Gospel of Matthew[5]

[32] After they had gone away, a demoniac who was mute was brought to him. [33] And when the demon had been cast out, the one who had been mute spoke; and the crowds were amazed and said, "Never has anything like this been seen in Israel." [34] But the Pharisees said, "By the ruler of the demons he casts out the demons."

## 4.2
## Jesus rejects conventional theodicies

*It was widely thought in the ancient world—and probably in most societies of all ages—that certain illnesses were punishment for sinful acts. This belief finds echoes in Mesopotamian theodicies, the book of Job, and Greek tragedy. It was held by many Jews and is found in the Gospels, where Jesus's disciples ask him whether the eighteen Galileans killed by a collapsing tower were punished for their sins or whether a man's congenital blindness was the result of his or someone else's sin. In both cases Jesus rejects this almost universally held popular explanation.*

### a. Jesus on illness as punishment for sin
Gospel of Luke[6]

13 At that very time there were some present who told him about the Galileans whose blood Pilate had mingled with their sacrifices. [2] He asked them, "Do you think that because these Galileans suffered in this way they were worse sinners than all other Galileans? [3] No, I tell you; but unless you repent, you will all perish as they did. [4] Or those eighteen who were killed when the tower of Siloam fell on them—do you think that they were worse offenders than all the others living in Jerusalem? [5] No, I tell you; but unless you repent, you will all perish just as they did."

### b. Jesus heals a blind man
Gospel of John[7]

9 As he walked along, he saw a man blind from birth. [2] His disciples asked him, "Rabbi, who sinned, this man or his parents, that he was born blind?" [3] Jesus answered, "Neither this man nor his parents sinned; he was born blind so that God's works might be revealed in him. [4] I must work the works of him who sent me while it is day; night is coming when no one can work. [5] As long as I am in the world, I am the light of the world." [6] When he had said this, he spat on the ground and made mud with the saliva and spread the mud on the man's eyes, [7] saying to him, "Go, wash in the pool of Siloam" (which means Sent). Then he went and washed and came back able to see. [8] The neighbors and those who had seen him before as a beggar began to ask, "Is this not the man who used to sit and beg?" [9] Some were saying,

"It is he." Others were saying, "No, but it is someone like him." He kept saying, "I am the man." [10] But they kept asking him, "Then how were your eyes opened?" [11] He answered, "The man called Jesus made mud, spread it on my eyes, and said to me, 'Go to Siloam and wash.' Then I went and washed and received my sight."

## 4.3
## Parable of the good Samaritan
### Gospel of Luke[8]

*The parable of the good Samaritan is found only in Luke's Gospel. It is given in response to the question asked of Jesus, "Who is my neighbor?" It is a striking example of Jesus's rejection of religious formalism, which requires mere outward obedience to the law, in favor of an emphasis on compassionate benevolence as evidence of true religion (cf. James 1:26). The priest and the Levite are religious figures who deliberately avoid the inconvenience of aiding a man in distress while the hated Samaritan, regarded as a half-breed and apostate, exhibits the compassion that is often emphasized in both Jewish piety and Jesus's teachings.*

[25] Just then a lawyer stood up to test Jesus. "Teacher," he said, "what must I do to inherit eternal life?" [26] He said to him, "What is written in the law? What do you read there?" [27] He answered, "You shall love the Lord your God with all your heart, and with all your soul, and with all your strength, and with all your mind; and your neighbor as yourself." [28] And he said to him, "You have given the right answer; do this, and you will live."

[29] But wanting to justify himself, he asked Jesus, "And who is my neighbor?" [30] Jesus replied, "A man was going down from Jerusalem to Jericho, and fell into the hands of robbers, who stripped him, beat him, and went away, leaving him half dead. [31] Now by chance a priest was going down that road; and when he saw him, he passed by on the other side. [32] So likewise a Levite, when he came to the place and saw him, passed by on the other side. [33] But a Samaritan while traveling came near him; and when he saw him, he was moved with pity. [34] He went to him and bandaged his wounds, having poured oil and wine on them. Then he put him on his own animal, brought him to an inn, and took care of him. [35] The next day he took out two denarii, gave them to the innkeeper, and said, 'Take care of him; and when I come back, I will repay you whatever more you spend.' [36] Which of these three, do

you think, was a neighbor to the man who fell into the hands of the robbers?" [37] He said, "The one who showed him mercy." Jesus said to him, "Go and do likewise."

## 4.4
## Jesus's disciples heal a lame man
### Acts of the Apostles[9]

*Jesus sometimes sent his disciples throughout Galilee on missions to preach, teach, and heal (see Luke 10:1–12). The book of Acts, which records the expansion of Christianity in the Mediterranean world, relates instances of miraculous healing by Jesus's disciples.*

3 One day Peter and John were going up to the temple at the hour of prayer, at three o'clock in the afternoon. [2] And a man lame from birth was being carried in. People would lay him daily at the gate of the temple called the Beautiful Gate so that he could ask for alms from those entering the temple. [3] When he saw Peter and John about to go into the temple, he asked them for alms. [4] Peter looked intently at him, as did John, and said, "Look at us." [5] And he fixed his attention on them, expecting to receive something from them. [6] But Peter said, "I have no silver or gold, but what I have I give you; in the name of Jesus Christ of Nazareth, stand up and walk." [7] And he took him by the right hand and raised him up; and immediately his feet and ankles were made strong. [8] Jumping up, he stood and began to walk, and he entered the temple with them, walking and leaping and praising God. [9] All the people saw him walking and praising God, [10] and they recognized him as the one who used to sit and ask for alms at the Beautiful Gate of the temple; and they were filled with wonder and amazement at what had happened to him.

## 4.5
## Healing by prayer and anointing

*Anointing for a variety of reasons was practiced by Jews (see Exodus 30:30; 1 Samuel 15:1). In the New Testament Gospels, it is sometimes used for healing (e.g., Mark 6:13). James establishes a rite of healing, though there is some ambiguity whether it is employed for a physical or a spiritual illness. The mention of a confession of sin perhaps indicates that the healing is intended for spiritual illnesses, and the prayers of the elders of the church are the focus of the first passage below. Epaphroditus was also healed when he was near death, apparently as the result of prayer. Both excerpts suggest that in the early Christian communities prayer and anointing complemented or accompanied ordinary healing by medicine.*

### a. Anointing for healing in the early church
Book of James[10]

[13] Are any among you suffering? They should pray. Are any cheerful? They should sing songs of praise. [14] Are any among you sick? They should call for the elders of the church and have them pray over them, anointing them with oil in the name of the Lord. [15] The prayer of faith will save the sick, and the Lord will raise them up; and anyone who has committed sins will be forgiven. [16] Therefore confess your sins to one another, and pray for one another, so that you may be healed. The prayer of the righteous is powerful and effective.

### b. Prayer for healing
Book of Philippians[11]

[25] Still, I think it necessary to send to you Epaphroditus—my brother and co-worker and fellow soldier, your messenger and minister to my need; [26] for he has been longing for all of you, and has been distressed because you heard that he was ill. [27] He was indeed so ill that he nearly died. But God had mercy on him, and not only on him but on me also, so that I would not have one sorrow after another. [28] I am the more eager to send him, therefore, in order that you may rejoice at seeing him again, and that I may be less anxious. [29] Welcome him then in the Lord with all joy, and honor such people, [30] because he came close to death for the work of Christ, risking his life to make up for those services that you could not give me.

### 4.6
### Unhealed illnesses in the New Testament

*The prominence given to Jesus's healing miracles in the Gospels has sometimes been taken to suggest that early Christians relied heavily on religious healing for their ills. But a close reading of the New Testament suggests that healing by natural means was employed and that not all believers were healed of their diseases. Although the New Testament frequently describes supernatural* or religious healing, it appears that early Christians continued to suffer from illness and, like their Jewish and pagan neighbors, they sought medical attention for them.

One finds in the New Testament cases of ordinary sickness, some of which were healed by medical means and some of which remained unhealed, which existed alongside sicknesses whose healing was attributed to prayer. Paul's "thorn in the flesh" is assumed to have been a physical ailment for which he prayed for delivery without receiving it. The New Testament epistles, which are intended to provide normative apostolic instruction to the churches, have little to say about physical healing. The emphasis in the early church was less on the healing of illness than on the endurance of suffering for its spiritual benefit and on the compassionate care of the sick.

### a. Paul's thorn in the flesh
Book of Corinthians[12]

Therefore, to keep me from being too elated, a thorn was given me in the flesh, a messenger of Satan to torment me, to keep me from being too elated. [8] Three times I appealed to the Lord about this, that it would leave me, [9] but he said to me, "My grace is sufficient for you, for power is made perfect in weakness." So, I will boast all the more gladly of my weaknesses, so that the power of Christ may dwell in me. [10] Therefore I am content with weaknesses, insults, hardships, persecutions, and calamities for the sake of Christ; for whenever I am weak, then I am strong.

### b. Paul's physical infirmity
Book of Galatians[13]

[13] You know that it was because of a physical infirmity that I first announced the gospel to you; [14] though my condition put you to the test, you did not scorn or despise me, but welcomed me as an angel of God, as Christ Jesus.

### c. Trophimus's illness
Book of Timothy[14]

Erastus remained in Corinth; Trophimus I left ill in Miletus.

# 4.7
## The Christian reception of Greek medicine

*In the second century Christianity attracted increasing numbers of educated Greeks, who had studied philosophy in Greek schools in the eastern Roman Empire. They were well read and had acquired the intellectual tools to defend Christian doctrines in a manner that could appeal to educated Greeks and Romans. They became known as apologists (from the word apologia, or "defense") for their ability to defend Christian ideas. Several were well read in medicine, which was a subject of study in Greek and Roman schools, and they valued its importance. They made it clear that educated Greeks and Romans, whether Christian or pagan, respected learned medicine and indeed employed it in treating illness. While their views of medicine varied, with some more critical than others, none of the apologists rejected medicine altogether, although Origen considered prayer to be superior to the use of medicine for healing, an approach that has remained a practice among some Christians ever since.*

### a. Biblical writers commend medicine
Tertullian, *de Corona*[15]

Let Æsculapius have been the first who sought and discovered cures: Isaiah mentions that he ordered Hezekiah medicine when he was sick. Paul, too, knows that a little wine does the stomach good.

### b. Pain is often required for medicine to heal
Tertullian, *Scorpiace* (adapted)[16]

This forwardness also appertains to men—to discard what is wholesome, to accept what is baleful, to avoid all dangerous cures, or, in short, to be eager to die rather than to be healed. For there are many who flee from the aid of physic also, many in folly, many from fear and false modesty. And the healing art has manifestly an apparent cruelty, by reason of the lancet, and of the burning iron, and of the great heat of the mustard; yet to be cut and burned, and pulled and bitten, is not on that account an evil, for it occasions helpful pains; nor will it be refused merely because it afflicts, but because it afflicts inevitably will it be applied. The good accruing is the apology for the frightfulness of the work. In short, that man who is howling and groaning and bellowing in the hands of a physician will presently load the same hands with a fee, and proclaim that they are the best operators, and no longer affirm that they are cruel.

### c. The existence of competing medical sects is no reason to deny the benefits of medicine
Origen, *Contra Celsum*[17]

To this we will reply that any teaching which has had a serious origin, and is beneficial to life, has caused different sects. For since medicine is beneficial and essential to mankind, and there are many problems in it as to the method of curing bodies, on this account several sects in medicine are admittedly found among the Greeks, and, I believe, also among the barbarians such as profess to practice medicine. . . . But the sects in medicine would be no good reason for avoiding it; nor would anyone who was endeavouring to act rightly hate philosophy, alleging the existence of many sects as an excuse for his hatred of it.

### d. Ordinary medicine and prayer provide two means of healing
Origen, *Contra Celsum*[18]

Even Celsus has to admit that they [daemons] can do nothing better than healing the body. However, I would affirm that it is not clear that these daemons, in whatever way they are worshipped, are even capable of healing bodies. A man ought to use medical means to heal his body if he aims to live in the simple and ordinary way. If he wishes to live in a way superior to that of the multitude, he should do this by devotion to the supreme God and by praying to Him.

### 4.8
### The Decian plague in Alexandria
Eusebius, *Ecclesiastical History*[19]

*Although Christianity had spread throughout the Roman Empire by the third century, Christians continued to face occasional and sporadic persecution until 313 CE. In 249 Emperor Decius ordered all imperial subjects to offer sacrifices to the pagan gods upon pain of death for those who refused. An epidemic broke out during this period of intense persecution, and Dionysius, the bishop*

*of Alexandria, Egypt, from 247 to 264, organized Christians in the city to un-*
*dertake systematic relief efforts on behalf of the plague victims. Eusebius pre-*
*served his letter that describes the plague.*

Later, when a severe epidemic followed the war just as the [Easter] festival
was approaching, he again communicated in writing with the Christian
community, revealing the horrors of the disaster:

Other people would not think this a time for festival: they do not so regard this or any other time, even if, so far from being a time of distress, it is
a time of unimaginable joy. Now, alas! all is lamentation, everyone in mourning, and the city resounds with weeping because of the number that have
died and are dying every day. As Scripture says of the firstborn of the Egyptians, so now there has been a great cry: there is not a house in which there
is not one dead—how I wish it had been only one!

Many terrible things had happened to us even before this. First we were
set on and surrounded by persecutors and murderers, yet we were the only
ones to keep festival even then. Every spot where we were attacked became
for us a place for celebrations, whether field, desert, ship, inn, or prison.
The most brilliant festival of all was kept by the fulfilled martyrs, who were
feasted in heaven. After that came war and famine, which struck at Christian and heathen alike. We alone had to bear the injuries they did us, but we
profited by what they did to each other and suffered at each other's hands;
so yet again we found joy in the peace which Christ has given to us alone.
But when both we and they had been allowed a tiny breathing-space, out of
the blue came this disease, a thing more terrifying to them than any terror,
more frightful than any disaster whatever, and as a historian of their own
[Thucydides, *History* 2.64.1] once wrote: "the only thing of all that surpassed
expectation." To us it was not that, but a schooling and testing as valuable as
all our earlier trials; for it did not pass over us, though its full impact fell on
the heathen. . . .

Most of our brother-Christians showed unbounded love and loyalty,
never sparing themselves and thinking only of one another. Heedless of the
danger, they took charge of the sick, attending to their every need and min-
istering to them in Christ, and with them departed this life serenely happy;
for they were infected by others with the disease, drawing on themselves
the sickness of their neighbours and cheerfully accepting their pains. Many,
in nursing and curing others, transferred their death to themselves and
died in their stead, turning the common formula that is normally an empty

courtesy into a reality: "Your humble servant bids you good-bye." The best of our brothers lost their lives in this manner, a number of presbyters, deacons, and laymen winning high commendation, so that death in this form, the result of great piety and strong faith, seems in every way the equal of martyrdom. With willing hands they raised the bodies of the saints to their bosoms; they closed their eyes and mouths, carried them on their shoulders, and laid them out; they clung to them, embraced them, washed them, and wrapped them in grave-clothes. Very soon the same services were done for them, since those left behind were constantly following those gone before.

The heathen behaved in the very opposite way. At the first onset of the disease, they pushed the sufferers away and fled from their dearest, throwing them into the roads before they were dead and treating unburied corpses as dirt, hoping thereby to avert the spread and contagion of the fatal disease; but do what they might, they found it difficult to escape.

### 4.9
### The plague in Carthage
Cyprian, *de Mortalitate*[20]

*The Decian plague spread from east to west, across North Africa to Carthage in 252 and then to Rome. Cyprian was the bishop of Carthage and an influential theologian and Christian leader. In his treatise* de Mortalitate *(On Death), Cyprian called on the Christians at Carthage not to fear death but to aid their persecutors during the plague and, in spite of the danger to themselves, to undertake the systematic care of the sick throughout the entire city. He urged them to make no distinction and minister to both Christians and pagans.*

But nevertheless it disturbs some that the power of this disease attacks our people equally with the heathen, as if the Christian believed for this purpose, that he might have the enjoyment of the world and this life free from the contact of ills; and not as one who undergoes all adverse things here and is reserved for future joy. It disturbs some that this mortality is common to us with others; and yet what is there in this world which is not common to us with others, so long as this flesh of ours still remains, according to the law of our first birth, common to us with them? So long as we are here in the world, we are associated with the human race in fleshly equality, but are separated in spirit. Therefore until this corruptible shall put on incorruption, and this mortal receive immortality, and the Spirit lead us to God the Father, whatsoever are the disadvantages of the flesh are common to us with the human race. Thus, when the earth is barren with an unproductive harvest, famine makes no distinction; thus, when with the invasion of an enemy any city is taken, captivity at once desolates all; and when the serene clouds withhold the rain, the drought is alike to all; and when the jagged rocks rend the ship, the shipwreck is common without exception to all that sail in her; and the disease of the eyes, and the attack of fevers, and the feebleness of all the limbs is common to us with others, so long as this common flesh of ours is borne by us in the world.

And further, beloved brethren, what is it, what a great thing is it, how pertinent, how necessary, that pestilence and plague which seems horrible and deadly, searches out the righteousness of each one, and examines the minds of the human race, to see whether they who are in health tend the sick; whether relations affectionately love their kindred; whether masters pity their languishing servants; whether physicians do not forsake the beseeching patients; whether the fierce suppress their violence; whether the rapacious can quench the ever insatiable ardour of their raging avarice even by the fear of death; whether the haughty bend their neck; whether the wicked soften their boldness; whether, when their dear ones perish, the rich, even then bestow anything, and give, when they are to die without heirs. Even although this mortality conferred nothing else, it has done this benefit to Christians and to God's servants that we begin gladly to desire martyrdom as we learn not to fear death. These are trainings for us, not deaths: they give the mind the glory of fortitude; by contempt of death they prepare for the crown.

## 4.10
## A late Roman plague
Eusebius, *Ecclesiastical History*[21]

*Eusebius vividly described a plague in the eastern Roman Empire that broke out in 312–13 CE during the reign of Maximin Daia, following a drought-induced famine while Christians were undergoing persecution. Because the government lacked any program for dealing with the crisis, there was no relief, and people were left to fend for themselves. The only care of the sick and dying was provided by Christian churches, which hired gravediggers to bury the dead.*

It was the winter season, and the usual rains and showers were withholding their normal downpour, when without warning famine struck, followed by pestilence and an outbreak of a different disease—a malignant pustule, which because of its fiery appearance was known as a carbuncle. This spread over the entire body causing great danger to the sufferers; but the eyes were the chief target for attack, and hundreds of men, women, and children lost their sight through it. . . . In the Armenian war the emperor was worn out as completely as his legions: the rest of the people in the cities under his rule were so horribly wasted by famine and pestilence that a single measure of wheat fetched 2,500 Attic drachmas. Hundreds were dying in the cities, still more in the country villages, so the rural registers which once contained so many names now suffered almost complete obliteration; for at one stroke food shortages and epidemic disease destroyed nearly all the inhabitants. . . .

Some people, shrunken like ghosts and at death's door, tottered and slipped about in all directions till, unable to stand, they fell to the ground; and as they lay face down in the middle of the streets, they implored passers-by to hand them a tiny scrap of bread, and with their life at its last gasp they called out that they were hungry—anything else than this anguished cry was beyond their strength. Others—men classed as well-to-do—were astounded by the number of beggars, and after giving to scores, they adopted for the future a hard and merciless attitude, in the expectation that very soon they themselves would be no better off; so that in the middle of public squares and narrow streets dead and naked bodies lay about unburied for days on end, furnishing a most distressing sight to all who saw them. Indeed some even became food for dogs, and it was mainly for this reason that the survivors turned to killing the dogs, for fear they might go mad and begin devouring human flesh. No less terrible was the pestilence which consumed every household, particularly those which were so well off for food that famine could not wipe them out. Men of great wealth, rulers, governors, and numberless officials, left by the famine to the epidemic disease as if on purpose, met a sudden and very swift end. Lamentations filled the air on every side, and in all the lanes, squares, and streets there was nothing to be seen except processions of mourners with the usual flute-playing and beating of breasts. In this way death wages war with these two weapons of pestilence and famine, swallowing whole families in a few moments, so that two or three dead bodies could be seen carried to the graveyard by a single group of mourners.

Such was the reward for Maximin's loud boasts and the cities' resolutions against us [Christians], while the fruits of the Christians' limitless enthusiasm and devotion became evident to all the heathen. Alone in the midst of this terrible calamity they proved by visible deeds their sympathy and humanity. All day long some continued without rest to tend the dying and bury them—the number was immense, and there was no one to see them; others rounded up the huge number who had been reduced to scarecrows all over the city and distributed loaves to them all, so that their praises were sung on every side, and all men glorified the God of the Christians and owned that they alone were pious and truly religious: did not their actions speak for themselves?

## 4.11
### Ephraim sets up a temporary hospital in Edessa
Sozomen, *Ecclesiastical History*[22]

*Sixty years after the famine and plague of Maximin, a similar famine occurred in the Syrian town of Edessa in 373. When the leaders of the city seemed to be without a plan to deal with the emergency, Ephraim (c. 306–373 CE), a deacon and an ascetic, took the initiative to set up three hundred beds in public porticoes to care for those who were suffering the effects of famine, both citizens and foreigners. (It was unusual in classical philanthropy to offer municipal benefits to foreigners.) His personal reputation was such that he was entrusted by the wealthy with funds to do this work. After a month of personally caring for the sick people, he died.*

The city of Edessa being severely visited by famine, he [Ephraim] quitted the solitary cell in which he pursued philosophy, and rebuked the rich for permitting the poor to die around them, instead of imparting to them of their superfluities; and he represented to them by his philosophy, that the wealth which they were treasuring up so carefully would turn to their own condemnation, and to the ruin of the soul, which is of more value than all riches, and the body itself and all other values, and he proved that they were putting no estimate upon their souls, because of their actions. The rich men, revering the man and his words, replied, We are not intent upon hoarding our wealth, but we know of no one to whom we can confide the distribution of our goods, for all are prone to seek after lucre, and to betray the trust placed in them. What think you of me? asked Ephraim. On their admitting that they considered him an efficient, excellent, and good man, and worthy, and that he was exactly what his reputation confirmed, he offered to undertake the distribution of their alms. As soon as he received their money, he had about three hundred beds fitted up in the public porches; and here he tended those who were ill and suffering from the effects of the famine, whether they were foreigners or natives of the surrounding country. On the cessation of the famine he returned to the cell in which he had previously dwelt; and, after the lapse of a few days, he expired.

## 4.12
### Augustine's miracle narratives
### *a. Changing view of miracles*
Augustine, *Retractations*[23]

*Early in his life Augustine (354–430 CE) accepted the common opinion in Christian circles that miracles no longer occurred, having ended with the age of the apostles, a view he set forth in de* Vera religione *(On True Religion). Later, he began to change his mind after some bones of the martyr Stephen, which were brought to Hippo in 424, allegedly wrought several miracles. The discovery of the bones of the martyrs Protasius and Gervasius shortly thereafter supposedly effected seventy miracles in less than two years. Augustine described his change of mind in his* Retractations.

Likewise, this statement of mine is indeed true: "These miracles were not allowed to last until our times lest the soul ever seek visible things whose novelty enkindled it." For not even now, when a hand is laid on the baptized, do they receive the Holy Spirit in such a way that they speak with the tongues of all nations; nor are the sick now healed by the passing shadow of the preachers of Christ. Even though such things happened at that time, manifestly these ceased later. But what I said is not to be so interpreted that no miracles are believed to be performed in the name of Christ at the present time. For, when I wrote that book, I myself had recently learned that a blind man had been restored to sight in Milan near the bodies of the martyrs in that very city, and I knew about some others, so numerous even in these times, that we cannot know about all of them nor enumerate those we know.

### *b. Discovery of the bones of Protasius and Gervasius*
Augustine, *Confessions*[24]

It was at that time that you made known to your servant whom I have named, where the bodies of Protasius and Gervasius, the martyrs, lay. You had kept them secretly stored uncorrupted in your hiding-place for many years, to bring them out at the proper time to check the imperial dowager's madness. With due honour they were dug up and transferred to Ambrose's basilica. Not only were those troubled by unclean spirits healed, as the evil presences confessed themselves, but a well-known citizen who had been many years blind, asked and heard the reason for the popular excitement. He jumped up and asked his guide to take him there. Led there he begged and won permission to touch with his handkerchief the casket of your saints, whose death is precious in your sight. He did this, placed it to his eyes, and they were immediately opened. Your praises glowed and shone as the fame of it spread. Thus the mind of that hostile woman, though not brought to the health of faith, was checked from its rage of persecution. Thanks to you, my God. Whence and whither have you led my memory that I should thus confess to you great things which I might have forgetfully passed over?

### c. The healing of Innocentius
Augustine, *The City of God*[25]

*Augustine became convinced that miracles of healing brought about by the discovery of the relics of martyrs were not sufficiently known, and he rebuked Christians who did not publicize their miraculous healings. He began to collect accounts of these healings, cataloging and publishing many of them in book 22 of* The City of God. *Most are cases of illness that were unsuccessfully treated by physicians. The interesting excerpt that follows is Augustine's description of the healing of the distinguished advocate Innocentius.*

But who but a very small number are aware of the cure which was wrought upon Innocentius, ex-advocate of the deputy prefecture, a cure wrought at Carthage, in my presence, and under my own eyes? For when I and my brother Alypius, who were not yet clergymen, though already servants of God, came from abroad, this man received us, and made us live with him, for he and all his household were devotedly pious. He was being treated by medical men for fistulae, of which he had a large number intricately seated in the rectum. He had already undergone an operation, and the surgeons were using every means at their command for his relief. In that operation he had suffered long-continued and acute pain; yet, among the many folds of the gut, one had escaped the operators so entirely, that, though they ought to have laid it open with the knife, they never touched it. And thus, though all those that had been opened were cured, this one remained as it was, and frustrated all their labour. The patient, having his suspicions awakened by the delay thus occasioned, and fearing greatly a second operation, which another medical man—one of his own domestics—had told him he must undergo, though this man had not even been allowed to witness the first operation, and had been banished from the house, and with difficulty allowed to come back to his enraged master's presence—the patient, I say, broke out to the surgeons, saying, "Are you going to cut me again? Are you, after all, to fulfil the prediction of that man whom you would not allow even to be present?" The surgeons laughed at the unskillful doctor, and soothed their patient's fears with fair words and promises. So several days passed, and yet nothing they tried did him good. Still they persisted in promising that they would cure that fistula by drugs, without the knife. They called in also another old practitioner of great repute in that department, Ammonius (for he was still alive at that time); and he, after examining the part, promised the same result as themselves from their care and skill. On this great authority, the patient became confident, and, as if already well, vented his good spirits in facetious remarks at the expense of his domestic physician, who had predicted a second operation. To make a long story short, after a number of days had thus uselessly elapsed, the surgeons, wearied and confused, had at last to confess that he could only be cured by the knife. Agitated with excessive fear, he was terrified, and grew pale with dread; and when he collected himself and was able to speak, he ordered them to go away and never to return. Worn out with weeping, and driven by necessity, it occurred to him to call in an Alexandrian, who was at that time esteemed a wonderfully skillful operator, that he might perform the operation his rage would not suffer them to do. But when he had come, and examined with a professional eye the traces of their careful work, he acted the part of a good man, and persuaded his patient to allow those same hands the satisfaction of finishing his cure which had begun it with a skill that excited his admiration, adding that there was no doubt this only hope of a cure was by an operation, but that it was thoroughly inconsistent with his nature to win the credit of the cure by doing the little that remained to be done, and rob of their reward men whose consummate skills, care, and diligence he could not but admire when he saw the traces of their work. They were therefore again received to favour; and it was agreed that, in the presence of the Alexandrian, they should operate on the fistula, which, by the consent of all, could now only be cured by the knife. The operation was deferred till the following day. But when they had left, there arose in the house such a wailing, in sympathy with the excessive despondency of the master, that it seemed to us like the mourning at a funeral, and we could scarcely repress it. . . . Whether the others prayed, and had not their attention wholly diverted by this conduct, I do not know. For myself, I could not pray at all. This only I briefly said in my heart: "O Lord, what prayers of Thy people dost thou hear if Thou hearest not these?" For it seemed to me that nothing could be added to this prayer, unless he expired in praying. We rose from our knees, and, receiving the blessing of the bishop, departed, the patient beseeching his visitors to be present next morning, they exhorting him to keep up his heart. The dreaded day dawned. The servants of God were present, as they had promised to be; the surgeons arrived; all that the circumstances required was ready; the frightful instruments are produced; all look on in wonder and suspense. While those who have most influence with the patient are cheering his fainting spirit, his limbs are arranged on the couch so as to suit the hand of the operator; the knots of the bandages are untied; the part is bared; the surgeon examines it, and, with knife in hand, eagerly looks for the sinus that is to be cut. He searches for it with his eyes; he feels for it with his finger; he applies every kind of scrutiny: he finds a perfectly firm cicatrix! No words of mine can describe the joy, and praise, and thanksgiving to the merciful and almighty God which was poured from the lips of all, with tears of gladness. Let the scene be imagined rather than described!

## 4.13
### Anthony heals a young woman
Athanasius, *Life of Anthony*[26]

*Athanasius wrote in Greek a biography of Anthony (251–356 CE), who was the founder of anchoritic (hermitic) monasticism in Egypt, shortly after Anthony's death. It was translated into Latin and became enormously popular, creating a new genre of literature known as "hagiography." Written accounts of the lives of saints described the miraculous exploits that were attributed to their subjects, including exorcism, miraculous healing, and even raising the dead. In late antiquity some monks enjoyed popularity as miracle workers in the eastern Roman Empire, whereas in the West miracles were generally associated with relics and tombs. Anthony became a Christian at the age of 20, adopted* an ascetic regimen, and withdrew into the desert. He lived to be 105, achieving legendary status in his own lifetime. In the following story by Athanasius, he is called Antony.

There was also a maiden from Busiris Tripolitana, who had a terrible and very hideous disorder. For the runnings of her eyes, nose, and ears fell to the ground and immediately became worms. She was paralysed also and squinted. Her parents having heard of monks going to Antony, and believing on the Lord who healed the woman with the issue of blood, asked to be allowed, together with their daughter, to journey with them. And when they received them, the parents together with the girl remained outside the mountain with Paphnutius, the confessor and monk; but the monks went in to Antony. And when they only wished to tell about the damsel, he anticipated them, and detailed both the sufferings of the child and how she journeyed with them. Then when they asked that she should be admitted, Antony did not allow it, but said, "Go, and if she be not dead, you will find her healed: for the accomplishment of this is not mine, that she should come to me, wretched man that I am, but her healing is the work of the Savior, who in every place shows His pity to them that call upon Him. Wherefore the Lord has inclined to her as she prayed, and His loving-kindness has declared to me that He will heal the child where she now is." So the wonder took place; and going out they found the parents rejoicing and the girl whole.

## 4.14
### Loving the sick poor
Gregory of Nyssa, *de Pauperibus amandis* 2[27]

*Gregory of Nyssa (c. 330–c. 395 CE), Basil of Caesarea (330–379 CE), and Gregory of Nazianzus (329–389 CE) were Cappadocian fathers who gave a new definition in Christian thought to the poor as people who shared in the divine image (imago Dei) because in their suffering they shared the suffering of Christ. They maintained that even the diseased body of a leper was sanctified by bearing the image of the savior, who had also suffered for humankind. This is the theme of Gregory of Nyssa's second sermon called de Pauperibus amandis (On Loving the Poor), composed between 372 and 382 CE, which helped to shape Christian attitudes to leprosy and the care of sick poor people. He regarded lepers not as repulsive creatures, but as those who bring holiness and healing from spiritual diseases to the physically healthy but spiritually needy who touch them. This view of human solidarity is grounded in the doctrine of the incarnation, which unites the human race with God and provides a basis for the compassionate care of those in need.*

What brings release from such fears? Choosing that way of life which the Word has just shown us, the truly fresh and living way. And what is this way? "I was hungry, I was thirsty, I was a stranger and naked, and sick, and in prison." "As much as you have done for one of these, you have done for me." And because of this, He says, "Come, blessed of my Father" (Matt. 25:35–40). And what do we learn from these words? That attention paid to the commandments is a blessing, but indifference to the commandments is condemnation. Let us love the blessing and flee the curse. It is for us on our own authority to choose or not to choose one of [these paths]. We will be in that place to which we incline with our will. Therefore, let us make the Lord of blessing our own Lord, the one who counts concern for those in need as concern for Himself.

We should do this especially now when the commandment takes much more substance according to the present condition of life when many are in need of necessities, but many are also in need regarding their own bodies, people who have been wasted away by this terrible disease [i.e., leprosy]. Thus, in concern for these victims, let us fulfill for ourselves the good command of love. . . .

This man, on the other hand, as though his nature has been altered, appears as something different, not the living being he was accustomed to be. His hands have taken up the function of feet; his knees have become his supports [on the ground]. The supports given him by nature (his feet) and his ankles have either fallen away completely or are hanging haphazardly and are dragged along according to the situation in the manner of small boats, pulled along by the side [of a larger ship]. Thus, when you see a man in such circumstances, do you not feel regard for your common relationship? Do you not have mercy on a being of your own race, or do you feel revulsion at his misfortune, and hate the supplicant and flee his approach as though it were the assault of a wild beast? And yet it would be well for you to consider carefully that an angel has taken hold of you, a man; and that [this] angel, though without a body or any material nature, felt no disgust at one who was mixed with flesh and blood. . . .

What is it, then, that we hear them say? How, without having committed any unjust deed, they were rejected by those who bore them; how they were driven out of cities, driven out of common associations, of feasts, and of festivals, like some murderers or those who kill their own fathers, condemned to perpetual flight. But they are far more unfortunate than these [criminals]. Indeed, it is possible for murderers to migrate somewhere else and live among men. These people, however, alone of all others, are rejected everywhere as though declared to be common enemies to all men. They are considered worthy of no shelter, of sharing no common table, of using no [common] implements. . . .

Perhaps, however, someone will say that this command is good for later, but right now he must be wary of some contagion and of the infectious quality of the disease. So that he might not suffer something unwanted, he thinks that he must flee the approach of such as these. Such are his words, excuses, and inventions—some specious coverings for his indifference regarding the commands of God. This, however, is not the truth. No fear attaches to carrying out this command. Let no one treat evil with evil. How many can one see among those who from youth to old age are employed in caring for these sick and have not at all weakened the natural sound constitution of the body because of such efforts? Nor is it likely that this would be the case.

Whenever these types of [apparently contagious] diseases occur such as epidemic humoral fluxes or other diseases of such a type that they depend on some outside cause such as corrupt air or water, many people suspect that the diseases cross over from those already seized by the sickness to those who draw near. I, however, think that in this situation the ailment does not induce disease in the healthy person from contagion, but rather that a common flux of humors is responsible for the similarity of the disease in many cases. These others, however, believe that [this] disease has its origin by crossing over from those already stricken to other people. This ailment, however, is marked out in the patient when the internal structure of such a disease is established and the blood suffers a certain contamination by the admixture of corrupting humors.

It is possible to learn that [what I have outlined above] is the case from the following fact. Does any contagion of the stronger nature ever occur from those of good health to those who are sick, even if the healthy are most heavily involved in caring for them? This is not the case. It is thus not likely that in the contrary direction the ailment would transfer from those who are sick to those who are healthy. If, on the other hand, there is so much gain from the commandment that the kingdom of heaven is prepared by fulfilling it, and on the other hand, there exists no harm to the body of the one who cares [for the sick], what is it, then, that prevents this command of love from being realized?

## 4.15
## Basil founds the first hospital
Gregory of Nazianzus, *Funeral Oration of Basil the Great*[28]

*Basil the Great was one of the Cappadocians whose interest in the poor led him to distribute food during a famine that broke out around 368–69 CE in Caesarea (modern Turkey), where he was bishop. About 372 he founded the first known hospital, which he called a poorhouse (ptochotropheion), but which became known as the Basileias (named after him). Created initially as a leprosarium, it had sections for six groups: the poor, the homeless and strangers, orphans and foundlings, lepers, the aged and infirm, and the sick. It was described in glowing terms by Gregory of Nazianzus in his funeral oration of Basil.*

35. He gathered together the victims of the famine with some who were but slightly recovering from it, men and women, infants, old men, every age which was in distress, and obtaining contributions of all sorts of food which can relieve famine, set before them basins of soup and such meat as was found preserved among us, on which the poor live. Then, imitating the ministry of Christ Who, girded with a towel, did not disdain to wash the disciples' feet, using for this purpose the aid of his own servants, and also of his fellow servants, he attended to the bodies and souls of those who needed it, combining personal respect with the supply of their necessity, and so giving them a double relief.

. . .

63. A noble thing is philanthropy, and the support of the poor, and the assistance of human weakness. Go forth a little way from the city and behold the new city, the storehouse of piety, the common treasury of the wealthy, in which the superfluities of their wealth, aye, and even their necessaries, are stored, in consequence of his exhortations, freed from the power of the moth, no longer gladdening the eyes of the thief, and escaping both the emulation of envy and the corruption of time: where disease is regarded in a religious light, and disaster is thought a blessing, and sympathy is put to the test. Why should I compare with this work Thebes of the seven portals, and the Egyptian Thebes, and the walls of Babylon, and the Carian tomb of Mausolus, and the Pyramids, and the bronze without weight of the

Colossus, or the size and beauty of shrines that are no more, and all the other objects of men's wonder, and historic record, from which their founders gained no advantage, except a slight reward of fame. My subject is the most wonderful of all, the short road to salvation, the easiest ascent to heaven. There is no longer before our eyes that terrible and piteous spectacle of men who are living corpses, the greater part of whose limbs have mortified, driven away from their cities and homes and public places and fountains, aye, and from their own dearest ones, recognizable by their names rather than by their features: they are no longer brought before us at our gatherings and meetings, in our common intercourse and union, no longer the objects of hatred, instead of pity on account of their disease; composers of piteous songs, if any of them have their voice still left to them. Why should I try to express in tragic style all our experiences, when no language can be adequate to their hard lot? He however it was, who took the lead in pressing upon those who were men, that they ought not to despise their fellowmen, nor to dishonour Christ, the one Head of all, by their inhuman treatment of them; but to use the misfortunes of others as an opportunity of firmly establishing their own lot, and to lend to God that mercy of which they stand in need at His hands. He did not therefore disdain to honour with his lips this disease, noble and of noble ancestry and brilliant reputation though he was, but saluted them as brethren, not, as some might suppose, from vainglory, (for who was so far removed from this feeling?) but taking the lead in approaching to tend them, as a consequence of his philosophy, and so giving not only a speaking, but also a silent, instruction. The effect produced is to be seen not only in the city, but in the country and beyond, and even the leaders of society have vied with one another in their philanthropy and magnanimity towards them. Others have had their cooks, and splendid tables, and the devices and dainties of confectioners, and exquisite carriages, and soft, flowing robes; Basil's care was for the sick, and the relief of their wounds, and the imitation of Christ, by cleansing leprosy, not by a word, but in deed.

## 4.16
### Fabiola founds a hospital in Rome
Jerome, *Epistles*[29]

*Following Basil's founding of the Basileias, which he placed in a monastic structure, hospitals rapidly expanded throughout the eastern Roman Empire*

*in the late fourth and fifth centuries, with bishops taking the initiative in found-*
*ing them. Hospitals spread to the western part of the empire a generation later.*
*The earliest was established in Rome about 390 by Fabiola, a noblewoman who*
*used her own funds to build the hospital and worked there herself. She gathered*
*poor sick people from public squares and personally nursed many of them. Her*
*friend Jerome described her hospital, which, he wrote, enjoyed such success*
*that within a year after its founding it was known from Parthia to Britain.*

Restored to communion before the eyes of the whole church, what did she
do? In the day of prosperity she was not forgetful of affliction; and, having
once suffered shipwreck she was unwilling again to face the risks of the sea.
Instead therefore of re-embarking on her old life, she broke up and sold all
that she could lay hands on of her property (it was large and suitable to her
rank), and turning it into money she laid out this for the benefit of the
poor. She was the first person to found a hospital, into which she might
gather sufferers out of the streets, and where she might nurse the unfortunate victims of sickness and want. Need I now recount the various ailments
of human beings? Need I speak of noses slit, eyes put out, feet half burnt,
hands covered with sores? Or of limbs dropsical and atrophied? Or of diseased flesh alive with worms? Often did she carry on her own shoulders
persons infected with jaundice or with filth. Often too did she wash away
the matter discharged from wounds which others, even though men, could
not bear to look at. She gave food to her patients with her own hand, and
moistened the scarce breathing lips of the dying with sips of liquid. I know
of many wealthy and devout persons who, unable to overcome their natural
repugnance to such sights, perform this work of mercy by the agency of
others, giving money instead of personal aid. I do not blame them and am
far from construing their weakness of resolution into a want of faith. While
however I pardon such squeamishness, I extol to the skies the enthusiastic
zeal of a mind that is above it. A great faith makes little of such trifles. But I
know how terrible was the retribution which fell upon the proud mind of
the rich man clothed in purple for not having helped Lazarus. The poor
wretch whom we despise, whom we cannot so much as look at, and the very
sight of whom turns our stomachs, is human like ourselves, is made of the
same clay as we are, is formed out of the same elements. All that he suffers
we too may suffer. Let us then regard his wounds as though they were our
own, and then all our insensibility to another's suffering will give way before
our pity for ourselves.

Not with a hundred tongues or throat of bronze could I exhaust the forms of fell disease which Fabiola so wonderfully alleviated in the suffering poor that many of the healthy fell to envying the sick. However she showed the same liberality towards the clergy and monks and virgins. Was there a monastery which was not supported by Fabiola's wealth? Was there a naked or bedridden person who was not clothed with garments supplied by her? Were there ever any in want to whom she failed to give a quick and unhesitating supply? Even Rome was not wide enough for her pity. Either in her own person or else through the agency of reverend and trustworthy men she went from island to island and carried her bounty not only round the Etruscan Sea, but throughout the district of the Volscians, as it stands along those secluded and winding shores where communities of monks are to be found.

## 4.17
## Letter from Julian to Arsacius
Julian, *Letters*[30]

*In 361 Constantine's nephew Julian ascended the throne. Raised a Christian, Julian renounced that faith as an adult and returned to paganism. He tried to organize paganism in an institutional model that imitated the Christian churches. In 362, in a letter to Arsacius, he urged the chief priest of Galatia in Asia Minor to establish pagan charitable foundations in every city for those in need. The tone of the letter makes it clear that the request was intended to capture the philanthropic initiative from the Christians. Julian was killed in battle in 363, and his plans were never realized.*

The Hellenic [pagan] religion does not yet prosper as I desire, and it is the fault of those who profess it; for the worship of the gods is on a splendid and magnificent scale, surpassing every prayer and every hope. May Adrasteia pardon my words, for indeed no one, a little while ago, would have ventured even to pray for a change of such a sort or so complete within so short a time. Why, then, do we think that this is enough, why do we not observe that it is their benevolence to strangers, their care for the graves of the dead and the pretended holiness of their lives that have done most to increase atheism [i.e., Christianity]? I believe that we ought really and truly to practice every one of these virtues. And it is not enough for you alone to practice them, but so must all the priests in Galatia, without exception. Either shame or persuade them into righteousness or else remove them from their priestly office, if they do not, together with their wives, children and servants, attend the worship of the gods but allow their servants or sons or wives to show impiety towards the gods and honour atheism more than piety. In the second place, admonish them that no priest may enter a theatre or drink in a tavern or control any craft or trade that is base and not respectable. Honour those who obey you, but those who disobey, expel from office. In every city establish frequent hostels in order that strangers may profit by our benevolence; I do not mean for our own people only, but for others also who are in need of money. I have but now made a plan by which you may be well provided for this; for I have given directions that 30,000 modii of corn shall be assigned every year for the whole of Galatia, and 60,000 pints of wine. I order that one-fifth of this be used for the poor who serve the priests, and the remainder be distributed by us to strangers and beggars. For it is disgraceful that, when no Jew ever has to beg, and the impious Galilaeans [i.e., Christians] support not only their own poor but ours as well, all men see that our people lack aid from us. Teach those of the Hellenic faith to contribute to public service of this sort, and the Hellenic villages to offer their first fruits to the gods; and accustom those who love the Hellenic religion to these good works by teaching them that this was our practice of old. At any rate Homer makes Eumaeus say: "Stranger, it is not lawful for me, not even though a baser man than you should come, to dishonour a stranger. For from Zeus come all strangers and beggars. And a gift, though small, is precious." Then let us not, by allowing others to outdo us in good works, disgrace by such remissness, or rather, utterly abandon, the reverence due to the gods. If I hear that you are carrying out these orders I shall be filled with joy.

## NOTES

1. Harnack, *Mission and Expansion of Christianity*, 1:19 5n1.
2. Luke 13:10–16.
3. Matthew 9:18–26.
4. Matthew 9:27–31.
5. Matthew 9:32–34.
6. Luke 13:1–5.
7. John 9:1–11.
8. Luke 10:25–37.
9. Acts 3:1–10.
10. James 5:13–16.
11. Philippians 2:25–30.

12. 2 Corinthians 12:7–10.

13. Galatians 4:13–14.

14. 2 Timothy 4:20.

15. Tertullian, *de Corona* 8.2, in Roberts and Donaldson, *Ante-Nicene Fathers*, http://www.tertullian.org/anf/anf03/anf03-10.htm#P1019_415012.

16. Tertullian, *Scorpiace* 5, ibid., http://www.tertullian.org/anf/anf03/anf03-45.htm #P10956_3079211.

17. Origen, *Contra Celsum*, trans. Henry Chadwick (Cambridge: Cambridge University Press, 1980), 3.12 (135–36). Reprinted with permission.

18. Ibid., 8.60 (498).

19. Eusebius, *Ecclesiastical History* 7.22, in Eusebius, *The History of the Church*, trans. G. A. Williamson (Harmondsworth, England: Penguin Books, 1965). Copyright © G. A. Williamson 1965. Reproduced by permission of Penguin Books Ltd.

20. Cyprian, *de Mortalitate* 8.8, 16, in Roberts et al., *Ante-Nicene Fathers*, 4:470–71, 473.

21. Eusebius, *Ecclesiastical History* 9.8, in Eusebius, *History of the Church*, 1–14.

22. Sozomen, *Ecclesiastical History* 3.16, in Schaff and Wace, *Nicene and Post-Nicene Fathers*, http://www.ccel.org/ccel/schaff/npnf202.iii.viii.xvi.html.

23. Augustine, *Retractations* 2.12.7 (55).

24. Augustine, *Confessions* 9.7 (222).

25. Augustine, *City of God* 22.8 (820–23).

26. Athanasius, *Life of Anthony* 58, in Schaff and Wace, *Nicene and Post-Nicene Fathers*, 4:1.

27. Gregory of Nyssa, *de Pauperibus amandis* 2, in Miller and Nesbitt, *Walking Corpses*, 175–84.

28. Gregory of Nazianzus, *Oration* 43.35, 63, in Schaff and Wace, *Nicene and Post-Nicene Fathers*, http://www.ccel.org/ccel/schaff/npnf207.iii.xxvi.html.

29. Jerome, *Letter* 77.6 (to Oceanus), ibid., http://www.ccel.org/ccel/schaff/npnf 206.v.LXIX.html.

30. Julian, *Letter* 49, in Julian, *Works of Emperor Julian*, 67–71.

# FIVE

# The Middle Ages

## INTRODUCTION

The question of the relationship between religion and medicine in the Middle Ages is vast and multivalent and, like all interdisciplinary investigations, may be approached through a multiplicity of intellectual entry points. Rather than employing a geographic or chronological approach, in this chapter I use a thematic organization. Given the limited boundaries of an anthology, this chapter does not include every theme pertaining to the intersection between medicine and religion during the Middle Ages. Rather, I highlight noteworthy texts providing representative examples of a range of major themes, questions, and concerns in religious engagements with disease, healing, and the work of physicians. Although these excerpts were produced in a variety of settings, in this chapter I pay particular attention to Christian engagements in the medieval West.

The period commonly defined by historians as the Middle Ages lasted from the fifth century CE (with the fall of the western Roman Empire in 476 CE generally treated as its starting point) to the mid- to late fifteenth century. This stage in the evolution of Western medicine is sometimes characterized as an age of "library medicine."[1] Formal medical education was based on studies of authoritative texts—rather than on experiments—especially those written by earlier Greek medical authors, such as Hippocrates and Galen, which were regarded as foundational. The Latin translation of the *Canon of Medicine*, originally composed by the Islamic scholar Avicenna (Ibn Sīnā), became an integral part of medical curricula after the mid-thirteenth century.

This long era displayed a remarkable continuity with earlier Christian history in the kinds of questions it engaged regarding religion and medicine. Among other things, writers addressed the occurrence and accessibility of supernatural healing, religious explanations of the meaning of illness, demonically caused disorders, and the boundaries of religiously acceptable healing practices. Yet at the same time, the Middle Ages provided a variety of changing contexts that significantly shaped the development of how medieval people both asked and sought to answer the earlier questions. A perceived need to carry out the ancient Christian moral imperative of caring for the sick resulted in the improvement of old organizational forms of medical charity and the establishment of new forms. People in the Middle Ages also transformed old religious practices for seeking healing and created a variety of new ones. A tradition of the devotional pursuit of physical suffering, largely associated with the mysticism of monastic women, developed during this era. Finally, a number of historically significant documents across religious traditions were produced that contributed to clarifying and defining norms for physicians' professional moral conduct.

Among such notable developments was the evolution of ideas about Christian sainthood, including the growing practice of seeking the help of saints in the struggle against physical maladies. The early medieval religious imagination was fascinated with the lives of so-called holy men and women. These deeply devout individuals pursued lives of virtue, prayer, and asceticism (in the East, commonly in the solitude of the desert) and reportedly performed miracles, including miracles of healing, for which they were frequently sought by suffering common folk. Furthermore, deceased saints gradually came to be seen as heavenly patrons able to help the living faithful, owing to the excess of spiritual merits their extraordinary righteousness had earned from God. Martyrs, ascetics, and notable church leaders were some of those in the heavenly ranks of saints, whose intercession was sought for physical recovery. Accounts of saints' lives were produced following the general conventions of a literary genre now referred to as "hagiography," or idealized biography. A hagiographic account combines informational history with semilegendary descriptions of a saint's miraculous deeds. A distinctly medieval theological development was the increased association of a saint's influence (and, consequently, his or her healing power) on earth with particular locations, objects, and, especially, his or her bodily remnants, which were believed to be physically incorruptible, owing to the presence of a special spiritual force.

An example of such religious sensibilities is recorded in *Life of St. Benedict* [5.1], a hagiography of the founder of Western monasticism, Benedict of Nursia, composed by Pope Gregory the Great in the late sixth century. The text narrates an episode of healing that miraculously occurred in Benedict's former dwelling cave, which is followed by a theological discussion that attributes healing powers to deceased saints. Such beliefs contributed to the flourishing of Christian pilgrimages to shrines hosting saints' relics with the purpose of securing healing. A later example of medieval hagiography from a different region is the eighth-century *Life of St. Cuthbert* [5.2] written by one of the most important intellectuals of his day, the Anglo-Saxon monk the Venerable Bede. This narrative also exhibits the medieval belief that a saint's healing power extended to material objects associated with him or her.

The seventh-century "Life of St. Theodore of Sykeon" [5.3] is an example of a hagiography, emerging from Eastern Christianity. The story links miraculous healing to an icon, which became a particular characteristic of Christian devotion in Orthodox Byzantium. From the early days of Christianity, differences gradually developed between certain expressions of Christian doctrine and practice, which distinguished the Roman Empire's predominantly Latin-speaking western part from its Greek-speaking eastern part. In contrast to the customs of the Latin West, images of Christ, Mary, and the saints acquired a special significance for Christian worship and devotion in what became the Greek Byzantine Empire. This significance did not go undisputed; however, after the iconoclastic controversy, the iconophiles ultimately won in 787. This outcome had a significant bearing on the relationship between religion and medicine in the Orthodox East. Icons became permanently viewed as emanating the special energies, including healing energies, of the holy people whose images they bore, and consequently, icons were understood to be agents of bodily healing. The resultant tradition of expressing physical devotion to the icons (viewed, at least ideally, as expressions of devotion to those whom the icons represented) included praying to, kneeling before, and kissing the icons, as the afflicted sought cures for their diseases.

As much as belief in supernatural healing was part of the Christian story from its beginning, dating back to biblical accounts of miraculous cures, so was the moral imperative to care self-sacrificially for the weak and vulnerable. In Matthew 25, Christ exhorts his followers to aid sick people as if they were Jesus himself struck by illness. The fulfillment of this ethical obligation was manifested in different forms in the Middle Ages. In addition to individual works of Christian charity, new forms of organized, religiously motivated medical service were developed. In the West, monasteries adopted an organizational structure that provided lodging for sick traveling pilgrims and needy poor people. The sixth-century Italian abbot St. Benedict of Nursia is regarded as the founder of a distinctly Western model of Christian monasticism. In contrast to the Byzantine asceticism of late antiquity, which was generally characterized by a solitary pursuit of holiness, Benedict emphasized the communal aspects of the monastic enterprise, in which life was to be centered on prayer and work. The Rule of St. Benedict [5.4] eventually became the model (and, until the twelfth century, the sole) order for Western monastic communities. Because Benedict's Rule articulated the special importance of the care of the sick, medical service became an integral part of medieval monasticism in the West. Starting in the twelfth century, mendicant orders and communities of pious laypeople dedicated to poverty and works of charity, such as the women's Beguine movement, became other vehicles of service to sick poor people, especially in growing urban areas.

In contrast to the West, Christian medical philanthropy in Byzantium was more of a joint effort between the church and the state. Originating in the fourth-century eastern Roman Empire as charitable Christian institutions, hospitals continued to grow in number in the Middle Ages and provided increasingly sophisticated medical care. The development of hospitals progressed more slowly in the medieval West. In the twelfth century, a military order of Hospitallers (Knights of St. John) operated a remarkably large and well-equipped hospital in Jerusalem dedicated to the service of poor people of all faiths. In the medieval Western imagination, this was an expectation-defying medical facility and an ideal model of Christian charitable enterprise. The medical work of Hospitallers was animated by the theological premise that poor sick people represented Christ and thus were to be rendered devoted service as if they were lords. Governed by the Rule of Raymond du Puy [5.5a], modeled after the Rule of St. Augustine, the order required from its members the renunciation of private property and a commitment to Christian moral standards of living. The Statutes of Roger des Moulins [5.5b] laid out the organization of the daily work of the Jerusalem hospital. The Jerusalem hospital also inspired the establishment of similarly organized, smaller institutions throughout Europe, especially as the increase of urban poverty due to growing urbanization in the thirteenth century made the need in the West acute.

From the twelfth century until the Reformation, Christian thought in western Christendom evolved in what can be described as three related yet distinct expressions: monastic, scholastic, and vernacular. The monastic tradition was largely concerned with devotional spirituality and piety, and it frequently engaged religious mysticism. The Christian religion had contained positive modes of conceptualizing suffering, including physical suffering, from its earliest days. However, in the context of medieval mystical monastic theological production and practice, especially as created and performed by women, the experience of bodily pain came to be sought and regarded as a profound devotional practice.[2] Such understandings of physical suffering were rooted in an ancient Christian imperative to be conformed to or to imitate Christ. Suffering was seen as a manifestation of such conformity, particularly with regard to Christ's Passion (the period from his agony in the garden of Gethsemane to the crucifixion). In the Middle Ages, religious imaginations came to emphasize the physical aspect of Jesus's Passion. Another theological underpinning of the medieval attraction to devotional physical suffering was a renewed emphasis on the relation of our humanity to the humanity of Christ, according to the Christian belief in the incarnation. Yet another religious basis for valorizing physical suffering was provided by interpreting the Pauline opposition of flesh and spirit as juxtaposing the physical and the spiritual aspects of being human. All these religious sensibilities were related to the flourishing interest—especially among women mystics—in the spiritual significance and implications of an active pursuit of bodily asceticism, mortifications, and experiences of other forms of pain and illness.

Such devotional interest in physical suffering characterized the writings of the fourteenth-century English mystic Julian of Norwich. An excerpt from her treatise *Showings* [5.6] portrays Julian's desire for illness and its subsequent occurrence as profound spiritual experiences. The extreme severity of the ascetic practices that spiritual medieval women were known to follow is illustrated by a biography of Julian's contemporary, the Italian lay Dominican mystic Catherine of Siena, written by her confessor Raymond of Capua. Raymond asserted that Catherine's radical asceticism and fasting had been unsurpassed in the history of the church. His *Life of St. Catherine of Siena* [5.7] claimed that physicians were unable to account for Catherine's continuous vitality despite her severe bodily mortifications and that Catherine's starving body was sustained contrary to the laws of nature by the "fullness" of her spirit.

As much as experiences of physical suffering were spiritually valorized and even pursued in certain medieval theological contexts, the disruptive and calamitous realities of pain, illness, and incapacitation continued to bring hardship and demanded both healing and religious interpretations. As faith in the reality of miraculous healings and a strong ethical imperative to care sacrificially for the sick characterized the Christian movement from the days of Jesus, so did quests for religious explanations of human suffering and death vis-à-vis a core Christian belief in a loving and merciful God. The death and sickness plaguing humanity came to be seen by Christians as an inherited consequence of Adam and Eve's fatal disobedience to God's commandment in the garden of Eden. That principal idea became foundational for many subsequent elaborate theological speculations about the origin and meaning of sickness and medicine. For instance, *Causes and Cures* [5.8], authored by the twelfth-century German Benedictine abbess Hildegard of Bingen, illustrates one such medieval religious exploration of the genesis, causes, and meanings of disease and healing. The treatise presented a mix of biblical teachings about the origin of human suffering and ideas current in Hildegard's own time regarding humoral medicine.

A recognized medical teacher and practitioner who also wrote extensively on practical methods of preventing and treating various illnesses, Hildegard lived at the end of the era of learned monastic medicine. In 1139, the Second Lateran Council [5.9] prohibited clergy from engaging in the study of jurisprudence and in the practice of medicine for the sake of material gain. The prohibition was not directed toward the long-standing tradition of religious medical charity, but rather was concerned with the clergy compromising their religious duties in order to make monetary profit. From the end of the twelfth century, universities gradually displaced monasteries as the centers of medical education. That displacement had implications for the participation in medicine of women like Hildegard: since universities were inaccessible to women, their perceived legitimacy as healers was significantly eroded.

The so-called scholastic theology was developed in university settings, where it was written and taught in Latin. Having been subjected to increased criticism in the late Middle Ages, scholastic theology experienced its golden age in the thirteenth century and the first half of the fourteenth. During this period gems of systematic Catholic theological treatises were created. These attempts to systematize medieval religious thought extended to questions of healing and physical suffering. Thomas Aquinas, a scholastic theologian, was arguably the most significant medieval Christian thinker. In his monumental treatise *Summa theologiae* [5.10], he sought to produce an organized synthesis of Christian teachings, or "sacred doctrine." Aquinas's method relied on theological premises revealed through faith and arguments derived from philosophical reasoning. Among its other explorations, the *Summa* contained discussions of questions pertaining to healing.

The academic exposition of "natural" versus "superstitious" in healing and sickness outlined by Aquinas, a renowned Dominican theologian, and his deployment of church tradition, particularly Augustinian, was later used by two Dominican inquisitors, Heinrich Krämer and Jacob Sprenger. These men authored one of the most infamous texts in the history of the church, *Malleus Maleficarum* (The Hammer of [Female] Witches) [5.11]. Published in the late Middle Ages, this manual for witch persecutors largely provided a program for more than two centuries of the European "witch craze" as well as for a religiously framed misogyny that was often deadly for its victims. It has been estimated that in the years following the publication of the manual, nearly 80 percent of those charged and executed for witchcraft were women.[3] *Malleus Maleficarum* maintained a traditional link between sudden and seemingly unexplainable physical maladies and the perceived activity of malicious sorceresses. Its striking recommendation to use the expertise of physicians in order to determine whether a person's sickness was caused by witches reminds contemporary readers of the porous boundaries between magic, "learned" medicine, and religion in the era of prescientific medicine.

Different cultures widely recognized the ability of physicians both to inflict significant harm and to accomplish much benefit. The task of defining moral expectations for a healer's professional conduct is an enterprise as old as the healing profession itself. In this endeavor, religion was frequently used to establish ethical guidelines for medical practices and to police their observance. Antoninus Pierozzi's *Summa theologica moralis* [5.12], written in the late Middle Ages as an aid to medieval confessors, contained occupation-specific descriptions of temptations and sins, including those characteristic of physicians. The restoration of a sinner to the state of grace, rather than punishment, was understood as the ultimate purpose of confession; through this idea of restoration, the labor of a confessor was likened to that of a physician. The important canon 21 of the Fourth Lateran Council [5.13a], which made the yearly practice of confession mandatory for all adult Catholic Christians, also instructed priests to imitate the work of skillful physicians in their diagnosis and treatment of human sin. Canon 22 [5.13b] of the same council in 1215 reaffirmed the superiority and precedence of spiritual over bodily healing and the traditional belief in a potential (albeit not necessary) connection between sin and disease. Therefore, physicians were to admonish seriously sick patients first to confess. They were also forbidden to recommend religiously illicit means of healing.

I conclude this chapter by looking at how religiously based expectations for medical practice were formulated within religious traditions other than Christianity during the Middle Ages. The seventh-century Chinese physician Sun Ssu-miao is commonly regarded as the founder of medical ethics in China, where the Hippocratic tradition was virtually unknown. His treatise *A Thousand Golden Remedies* [5.14] contained a discussion of medicine and the ethical obligations of physicians based on Taoist teachings; it was also likely influenced by Buddhist thought. In Judaism, the Oath of a Physician [5.15a], composed in the tradition of the Hippocratic Oath and attributed to the great twelfth-century Jewish thinker and physician Moses Maimonides, evoked the divine in the physician's commitment to upholding certain ethical guidelines. Finally, an excerpt from Maimonides's famed *Commentary on the Mishnah* [5.15b] provides an illustration from Judaism for the long-standing practice of drawing metaphorical parallels between physical and spiritual health and healing.

## TEXTS

### 5.1
### Religious healing in Western Christianity I: Saints and martyrs
Gregory the Great, *Life of St. Benedict*[4]

*St. Gregory the Great (540–604 CE) was a pope, writer, and civic administrator, who was subsequently recognized as one of the Latin fathers and a doctor of the church. Gregory abandoned his distinguished civic career as a prefect of Rome to become a monk, and eventually he ascended to the papacy in 590 as*

*Gregory I. According to tradition, Gregory was initially so reluctant to assume the burdens of the pontificate that he fled Rome, but in three days he was captured and brought back by the city's people, and he eventually relented. This excerpt is from the first biography of the founder of Western monasticism, St. Benedict of Nursia, which Gregory wrote based on the accounts received from four disciples of Benedict. This text appeared in about 593 in the second volume of Gregory's* Dialogues, *which is structured as conversations with his junior companion, Deacon Peter.*

In the cave of Subiaco where he had lived earlier, to this day dazzling miracles still occur if the faith of those who ask demands it. Recently something happened which I shall tell you about: a madwoman had lost her senses completely and was wandering night and day over mountains and through valleys, forests, and fields. She would only rest where exhaustion forced her to do so. One day when she was wandering without stopping, she came to the cave of that blessed man, father Benedict: she entered it and stayed there without realizing where she was. When morning came she departed, her mind restored to such perfect health that it was as if no madness had ever gripped her. For the rest of her life she continued in the same state of health which she had recovered there.

Peter: How is it that we often find the same thing happening in the case of the patronage of martyrs? They do not offer as much assistance through their bodily remains as through their relics and they perform greater miracles in those places where they are not actually buried?

Gregory: It is certain, Peter, that the holy martyrs can perform many marvels in those places where they are buried, as indeed they do, and reveal innumerable miracles to those who seek with a pure mind. But because it is possible that weak minds might doubt whether the holy martyrs are present and listening in those places where they are obviously not physically present, it is necessary for them to perform impressive miracles in those places where a weak mind might doubt their presence. But those whose mind is fixed in God gain greater merit for their faith, for they know that the martyrs are listening even though their bodies are not buried there.

## 5.2
# Religious healing in Western Christianity II: Healing objects
Bede, "Life of St. Cuthbert"[5]

*The Venerable Bede (673–735 CE) was an Anglo-Saxon monastic intellectual during the golden age of English monasticism and is regarded as the "father of English history." His "Life of St. Cuthbert" is a hagiographic account of one of the most popular medieval English miracle workers, the seventh-century bishop Cuthbert. According to tradition, in the early eighth century, Cuthbert's uncorrupted remains were found. This discovery energized devotion to him and prompted Bede to write his first hagiography of the saint. This excerpt is from the second, longer version of Bede's account of Cuthbert's life, which is based on an earlier, anonymously composed* Life of Cuthbert. *This passage tells the story of a pious abbess, Aelfflaed, and a nun being miraculously healed by a linen girdle or belt sent by Cuthbert.*

She {abbess Aelfflaed} had been seriously ill for a long time and seemed almost on the point of dying. The doctors could do nothing for her. By God's grace she was suddenly removed from danger of death though not entirely cured; the internal pain went and she regained the use of her limbs but still could not stand upright nor move about except on all fours. She began to fear that the condition might be permanent, since she had long since given up hope of getting any help from doctors. One day oppressed by these sad thoughts her mind wandered to the peaceful life Cuthbert led.

"How I wish I had something belonging to my dear Cuthbert!" she sighed. "As I trust and believe in God I know for certain that I should be quickly healed."

Shortly afterwards someone arrived with a linen cincture sent by Cuthbert. She was delighted with the gift and realized that her wishes had been made known to him by heavenly means. She girded herself with it and next morning was able to stand up straight. Two days later she was completely well. A few days after this one of the nuns was seized with excruciating pains in the head. She got daily worse until it seemed unlikely she could last much longer. The venerable abbess paid her a visit, saw how ill she was, and bound up her head with the cincture. The pain left her that very same day and she was cured.

## 5.3
### Religious healing in Eastern Christianity: Icons
*Life of St. Theodore of Sykeon*[6]

*St. Theodore the Sykeote (d. 613) was a Byzantine ascetic and the bishop of Anastasiopolis. According to a hagiography attributed to his disciple Eleusius, Theodore was born to a prostitute and an imperial messenger in the village of Sykeon in Galatia, Asia Minor. At the age of twelve, the boy was healed from the bubonic plague by a few drops of dew miraculously falling on him from an icon. Later, Theodore became known as a miracle worker, in particular for his gift of healing. The following excerpt from Theodore's hagiography focuses on another instance of miraculous healing involving an icon later in the saint's life.*

It happened that he fell so ill of a desperate sickness that he saw the holy angels coming down upon him; and he began to weep and to be sorely troubled. Now above him there stood an icon of the wonderworking saints Cosmas and Damian. These saints were seen by him looking just as they did in that sacred icon and they came close to him, as doctors usually do; they felt his pulse and said to each other that he was in a desperate state as his strength had failed and the angels had come down from heaven to him. And they began to question him saying, "Why are you weeping and are sore troubled, brother?" He answered them, "Because I am unrepentant, sirs, and also because of this little flock which is only newly instructed and is not yet stablished and requires much care." They asked him, "Would you wish us to go and plead for you that you may be allowed to live for a while?" He answered, "If you do this, you would do me a great service, by gaining for me time for repentance and you shall win the reward of my repentance and my work from henceforth." Then the saints turned to the angels and besought them to grant him yet a little time while they went to implore the King on his behalf. They agreed to wait. So the saints departed and entreated on his behalf the heavenly King, the Lord of life and death, Christ our God, Who granted unto Hezekiah the King an addition unto his life of fifteen years. They obtained their request and came back to the Saint bringing with them a very tall young man, like in appearance to the angels that were there, though differing from them greatly in glory. He said to the holy angels, "Depart from him, for supplication has been made for him to the Lord of all and King of glory, and He has consented that he should remain for a while in the flesh." Straightway both they and the young man disappeared from his sight, going up to heaven. But the Saints, Cosmas and Damian, said to the Saint, "Rise up brother, and look to thyself and to thy flock; for our merciful Master Who readily yields to supplication has received our petition on your behalf and grants you life."

## 5.4
## Caring for the sick in monasteries
### Benedict of Nursia, Rule of St. Benedict[7]

*St. Benedict of Nursia (c. 480–545 CE), an Italian monk and the founder of what later became known as the Benedictine monastic order, is commonly regarded as the father of Western monasticism. Benedict's career as an abbot allegedly had a difficult start: his first monks, frustrated by his strictness, attempted to poison his wine. Escaping the poison, Benedict went on to establish twelve monastic communities before founding his famous monastery on Monte Cassino. The seventy-three-chapter Rule of St. Benedict, written sometime after 530, laid out the order of administration, ethical principles, and rules for daily communal life at Monte Cassino. The monks vowed to observe obedience, the stability of place (permanent residency in a monastery), and the conversion of ways (radical life-style commitments), which included chastity and poverty. This excerpt from chapter 36 provided instructions regarding care for the sick.*

### Chapter 36. Sick brothers

The care of the sick must take precedence over everything else, so that they may be served just like Christ, for Christ said, "I was sick and you visited me" (Matt. 25:36) and "What you did for one of these, insignificant though they be, you did for me" (Matt. 25:40). For their part the sick should consider that they are being served out of reverence for God and must not irritate the brothers who are serving them by making unreasonable demands. One must, however, put up with them patiently because greater rewards are derived from people like this. The abbot should therefore take the greatest care that no one is neglected.

A special room should be assigned to brothers who are sick, together with someone to attend to them who is God-fearing, loving and attentive. The sick should be allowed to take a bath whenever necessary, but those who are healthy, especially the younger brothers, should only be allowed a bath occasionally. Those who are very weak should be allowed to eat meat to regain their strength, but when they are better they should abstain from meat as usual. The abbot should take the greatest care that the cellarers {chief stewards of the monastery} and attendants do not neglect the sick, for he is responsible for all the failures of his disciples.

## 5.5
## Medieval hospitals

*The Order of Hospitallers (Knights of St. John) was officially recognized by Pope Paschal II in 1113. The Hospitallers established and ran a hospital in Jerusalem that, according to contemporaries, boasted an impressive roster of nearly 150 people who worked there; held between a thousand and two thousand beds; and provided both medications and professional physicians' services. Serving sick poor people was the focus of the hospital's work.*

### a. Serving the sick poor
### The Rule of Raymond du Puy[8]

*This excerpt is from the instituting Rule of the order (the exact date of its first promulgation is unknown) written by its founder, Raymond du Puy.*

1. How The Brethren Should Make Their Profession: Firstly, I ordain that all the brethren, engaging in the service of the poor, should keep the three things with the aid of God which they have promised to God, that is to say, chastity and obedience, which means whatever thing is commanded them by their masters, and to live without property of their own: because God will require these three things of them at the Last Judgement.

2. What The Brethren Should Claim As Their Due: And let them not claim more as their due than bread and water and raiment, which things are promised to them. And their clothing should be humble, because Our Lord's poor, whose servants we confess ourselves to be, go naked. And it is a thing wrong and improper for the servant that he should be proud, and his Lord should be humble.

. . .

16. How Our Lords The Sick Should Be Received And Served: And in that obedience in which the master and the chapter of the Hospital shall permit, when the sick man shall come there, let him be received thus, let him partake

of the Holy Sacrament, first having confessed his sins to the priest, and afterwards let him be carried to bed, and there as if he were a Lord, each day before the brethren to eat, let him be refreshed with food charitably according to the ability of the House; also on every Sunday let the Epistle and the Gospel be chanted in that House, and let the House be sprinkled with holy water at the procession.

### b. Hospital organization
Statutes of Roger des Moulins[9]

*This excerpt is from statutes written around 1181 by Roger des Moulins, further outlining the theological and organizational principles for the order's service to sick poor people and for other charitable activities.*

2. And secondly, it is decreed with the assent of the brethren that for the sick in the Hospital of Jerusalem there should be engaged four wise doctors, who are qualified to examine urine, and to diagnose different diseases, and are able to administer appropriate medicines.

3. And thirdly, it is added that the beds of the sick should be made as long and as broad as is most convenient for repose, and that each bed should be covered with its own coverlet, and each bed should have its own special sheets.

4. After these needs is decreed the fourth command, that each of the sick should have a cloak of sheepskin and boots for going to and coming from the latrines, and caps of wool.

5. It is also decreed that little cradles should be made for the babies of the women pilgrims born in the House, so that they may lie separate, and that the baby in its own bed may be in no danger from [the] restlessness of its mother.

6. Afterwards it is decreed the sixth clause, that the biers of the dead should be concealed in the same manner as are the biers of the brethren, and should be covered with a red coverlet having a white cross.

7. The seventh clause commands that wheresoever there are hospitals for the sick, that the Commanders of the houses should serve the sick cheerfully, and should do their duty by them, and serve them without grumbling or complaining, so that by these good deeds they may deserve to have their reward in the glories of heaven. And if any of the brethren should act contrary to the commands of the Master in these matters, that it should be

brought to the notice of the Master, who shall punish them according to the sentence of the house commands.

. . .

10. Moreover guarding and watching them day and night, the brethren of the Hospital should serve the sick poor with zeal and devotion as if they were their lords, and it was added in Chapter-General that in every ward and place in the Hospital, nine sergeants should be kept at their service, who should wash their feet gently, and change their sheets, and make their beds, and administer to the weak necessary and strengthening food, and do their duty devotedly, and obey, in all things for the benefit of the sick.

The Confirmation by the Master Roger of the Things That the House Should Do: Let all the brethren of the House of the Hospital, both those present and those to come, know that the good customs of the House of the Hospital of Jerusalem are as follows:

1. Firstly the Holy House of the Hospital is accustomed to receive sick men and women, and is accustomed to keep doctors who have the care of the sick, and who make the syrups for the sick, and who provide the things that are necessary for the sick. For three days in the week the sick are accustomed to have fresh meat, either pork or mutton, and those who are unable to eat it have chicken.

2. And two sick persons are accustomed to have one coat of sheepskin which they use when going to the latrines, and between two sick persons one pair of boots. Every year the House of the Hospital is accustomed to give to the poor one thousand cloaks of thick lamb skins.

3. And all the children abandoned by their fathers and mothers the Hospital is accustomed to receive and to nourish. To a man and woman who desire to enter into matrimony, and who possess nothing with which to celebrate their marriage, the House of the Hospital is accustomed to give two bowls or the rations of two brethren.

4. And the House of the Hospital is accustomed to keep one brother shoemaker and three sergeants, who repair the old shoes given for the love of God. And the Almoner is accustomed to keep two sergeants who repair the old robes that he may give them to the poor.

5. And the Almoner [officer who administers alms] is accustomed to give twelve deniers to each prisoner, when he is first released from prison.

6. Every night five clerics are accustomed to read the Psalter for the benefactors of the House.

7. And every day thirty poor persons are accustomed to be fed at table once a day for the love of God, and the five clerics aforesaid may be among those thirty poor persons, but the twenty-five eat before the Convent, and each of the five clerics should have two deniers and eat with the Convent.

8. And on three days of the week they are accustomed to give in alms to all who come there to ask for it, bread and wine and cooked food.

9. In Lent every Saturday, they are accustomed to celebrate Maundy for thirteen poor persons, and to wash their feet, and to give to each a shirt and new breeches and new shoes, and to three chaplains, or to three clerics out of the thirteen, three deniers and to each of the others, two deniers.

10. These are the special charities decreed in the Hospital, apart from the Brethren-at-Arms whom the House should maintain honorably, and many other charities there are which cannot be set out in detail each one by itself. And that these things be true good men and loyal here bear witness, that is to say Brother Roger, Master of the Hospital, and Brother Bernard the Prior and all the Chapter-General.

## 5.6
## Illness and medieval Christian mysticism
Julian of Norwich, *Showings*[10]

*Julian of Norwich (c. 1342–c. 1416) was a Christian mystic and anchoress, who lived in religious seclusion in a cell adjoining the church at Norwich, England. She is the first known female author of a literary work in English. Julian became prominent for the expositions of sin, forgiveness, and prayer in her mystical writings, as well as for developing the theme of a motherly aspect of God within the Christian tradition. A devotional interest in physical suffering—both Jesus's physical torments and humans' bodily suffering as a way of imitating the incarnate God—was extremely important for Julian's theology. This excerpt is from the so-called long version of Julian's famous mystical treatise* Showings. *The treatise started with Julian's desire to experience what she described as three graces from God, the second of which, discussed here, was bodily sickness.*

As to the second grace, there came into my mind with contrition—a free gift which I did not seek—a desire of my will to have by God's gift a bodily sickness. I wished that sickness to be so severe that it might seem mortal, so that I might in it receive all the rites which Holy Church has to give me, whilst I myself should think that I was dying, and everyone who saw me would think the same; for I wanted no comfort from any human, earthly life in that sickness. I wanted to have every kind of pain, bodily and spiritual, which I should have if I had died, every fear and temptation from devils, and every other kind of pain except the departure of the spirit. I intended this because I wanted to be purged by God's mercy, and afterwards live more to his glory because of that sickness; because I hoped that this would be to my reward when I should die, because I desired soon to be with my God and my Creator. . . .

And when I was thirty and a half years old, God sent me a bodily sickness in which I lay for three days and three nights, and on the third night I received all the rites of Holy Church, and did not expect to live until day. And after this I lay for two days and two nights, and on the third night I often thought that I was on the point of death, and those who were with me often thought so. And yet in this I felt a great reluctance to die, not that there was anything on earth which it pleased me to live for, or any pain of which I was afraid, for I trusted in the mercy of God. But it was because I wanted to live for God better and longer, so that I might through the grace of that living have more knowledge and love of God in the bliss of heaven. Because it seemed to me that all the time that I had lived here was very little and short in comparison with the bliss which is everlasting, I thought: Good Lord, can my living no longer be to your glory? And I understood by my reason and the sensation of my pains that I should die; and with all the will of my heart I assented to be wholly as was God's will.

So I lasted until day, and by then my body was dead from the middle downwards, as it felt to me. Then I was helped to sit upright and supported, so that my heart might be more free to be at God's will, and so that I could think of him whilst my life would last. My curate was sent for to be present at my end; and before he came my eyes were fixed upwards, and I could not speak. He set the cross before my face, and said: I have brought the image of your savior; look at it and take comfort from it. It seemed to me that I was well, for my eyes were set upwards towards heaven, where I trusted that I by God's mercy was going; but nevertheless I agreed to fix my eyes on the face of the crucifix if I could, and so I did, for it seemed to me that I would hold out longer with my eyes set in front of me rather than upwards. After this my sight began to fail. It grew as dark around me in the room as if it had been night, except that there was ordinary light trained upon the image of the cross, I did not know how. Everything around the cross was ugly and terrifying to me, as if it were occupied by a great crowd of devils.

After this the upper part of my body began to die, until I could scarcely feel anything. My greatest pain was my shortness of breath and the ebbing of my life. Then truly I believed that I was at the point of death. And suddenly at that moment all my pain was taken from me, and I was as sound, particularly in the upper part of my body, as ever I was before. I was astonished by this sudden change, for it seemed to me that it was by God's secret doing and not natural; and even so, in this ease which I felt, I had no more confidence that I should live, nor was the ease I felt complete for me, for I thought that I would rather have been delivered of this world, because that was what my heart longed for.

**5.7**
### Religion and bodily mortifications
Raymond of Capua, *The Life of St. Catherine of Siena*[11]

*St. Catherine of Siena (1347–1380) was a lay Italian Dominican mystic. An important ecclesial political figure known for her holiness and works of charity, Catherine was involved in efforts to resolve political dissensions in Italy and is credited with having persuaded Pope Gregory XI to move the papal residence from Avignon back to Rome in 1377. Catherine was also known for her extreme asceticism and fasting. The following excerpt from her biography, written by her confessor, the Dominican friar Raymond of Capua, outlines some of her most rigid ascetic practices. In 1970, Catherine was given the title of doctor of the church, the second woman to receive such recognition in Roman Catholicism.*

When she {Catherine} was fifteen she gave up wine and drank nothing but well water. She also gradually learned to do without any kind of cooked food except bread, and soon reached the point of living entirely on bread and raw herbs. When she was about twenty, I think, she gave up eating bread altogether, and lived entirely on raw herbs. In the end it was given her, not as a result of habit or natural disposition, but as I hope, God willing, to explain more fully later, through a divine miracle, to reach such a point that though her wasted body was plagued by complaints and subject to labours that others would never have been able to endure, nevertheless the vital juices were not consumed within her; and though her stomach would not digest anything her physical powers were not at all enfeebled by this lack of food and drink. It always seemed to me that her whole life was a miracle, for what was visible before our eyes was something that could not possibly have taken place as the result of a natural process, as I was told plainly by the doctors I took to see her. But all these things, God willing, will be dealt with more fully later.

To end this part about her abstinence, you can rest assured, reader, that all the time I had the good fortune to be in Catherine's company she lived without eating or drinking, and endured unbearable pains and labours with an always joyful countenance without any help from nature. But it would be wrong to think that it was by any kind of effort or experience or habit of a natural kind that she reached this state or that anyone else could do such things. They were far too extraordinary for that, the result of fullness of spirit rather than any practice or habit of abstinence. As you know, fullness of spirit overflows into the body, because while the spirit is feeding the body finds it easier to endure the pangs of hunger. Can any Christian doubt this? Is it not a fact that the holy martyrs rejoiced in the torments of hunger in a quite unnatural way, as they did other bodily sufferings? How did they do this if not through fullness of spirit? I myself know from experience, and believe that anyone can prove it for himself, that while we are attending to God we find it easy to fast, but if we turn to other things we find it well-nigh impossible to go on with it. Why is this if not because in the former case the fullness of the spirit is sustaining the body with which it is hypostatically united? Such a thing may be above nature, but the body and spirit naturally communicate both good things and bad to each other. I do not deny that some people find it easier to fast than others; but I do not see how a fast can go on as long as Catherine's did on any natural basis. Let this suffice for the moment for the matter of the virgin's abstinence.

### 5.8
### Religious origins of disease
Hildegard of Bingen, *Causes and Cures*[12]

*Hildegard of Bingen (1098–1179) is the historically earliest woman to be recognized as a doctor of the church in Roman Catholicism (declared by Pope Benedict XVI in 2012). Hildegard was a German Benedictine abbess, mystical theologian, musician, medical practitioner, and prolific writer with a strong interest in medicine. Hildegard's medical theories were developed within the framework of humoral physiology, which was highly influential in the Middle Ages. Humoral medicine regarded a human body as containing four humors, the imbalance of which was believed to cause disease. The following excerpt from Hildegard's treatise* Causes and Cures *brings together medieval religious and humoral physiological teachings to offer an explanation of the origins of human illnesses, including melancholia (a medieval umbrella term for depressive and mood disorders). The terms* flegma *and* livor *are used by Hildegard to refer to, respectively, the predominant and secondary humors.*

That some people suffer from various infirmities stems from the *flegma* that abounds in them. For if the human had remained in Paradise he would not have in his body those *flegmata* leading to many evils but, rather, his flesh would be undamaged and without *livor.* When he consented to evil and relinquished good he was made similar to the earth that produces good and useful as well as bad and useless plants and that has good and bad moisture and sap within itself. With the taste for evil the blood of Adam's children was changed into the poison of semen from which the humans' offspring are propagated. Therefore their flesh is ulcerous and perforated. Those ulcers and perforations cause some kind of storm and a vaporous moisture in human beings. From this develop and coagulate *flegmata* that affect the human body with various infirmities. All of this arose from the first evil that a human first performed. Because had Adam remained in Paradise he would have had the sweetest health and the best dwelling, just as the strongest balsam gives off the best fragrance. But now, by contrast, human beings have poison in them, *flegma* and various infirmities. . . .

There are other persons who are sad and fearful and vacillate in their moods so that there exists no right disposition and state for them. They are like a strong wind that is useless for all plants and fruit. From this a *flegma* grows in them that is neither moist nor dense, but tepid. It is like *livor* that is tenacious and stretches like gum. It produces black bile that first originated from Adam's semen through the breath of the serpent, since Adam heeded its counsel in taking food. . . .

This black bile is dark and bitter and spews out every evil, sometimes even [causes] an infirmity of the brain. It lets the blood vessels of the heart bubble up, so to speak. It causes sadness and doubt about every kind of consolation, so that human beings can feel no joy about the heavenly life and can take no comfort in their present life. Through the Devil's first suggestion, when the human transgressed God's precept with the food of the apple, this melancholia belongs to the nature of every human being. From this food black bile developed in Adam and in his entire kind and rouses every plague in human beings.

## 5.9
## Ecclesial practice of medicine
### Second Lateran Council: Canon 9[13]

*The Second Lateran Council (the tenth ecumenical council) was called by Pope Innocent II in 1139. The following excerpt is from the council's canon 9, which prohibited clerics from studying and practicing civil law and medicine for the sake of financial gain and neglecting their religious duties.*

Moreover, the evil and detestable practice has grown, so we understand, whereby monks and canons regular, after receiving the habit and making their profession, are learning civil law and medicine with a view to temporal gain, in scornful disregard of the rules of their blessed teachers Benedict and Augustine. In fact, burning with the fire of avarice, they make themselves the advocates of suits; and since they have to neglect the psalmody and hymns, placing their trust in the power of fine rhetoric instead, they confuse what is right and what is wrong, justice and iniquity, by reason of the variety of their arguments. But the imperial constitutions testify that it is truly absurd and reprehensible for clerics to want to be experts in the disputes of law courts. We decree by apostolic authority that lawbreakers of this kind are to be severely punished. There are also those who, neglecting the care of souls, completely ignore their state in life, promise health in return for hateful money and make themselves healers of human bodies. And since an immodest eye manifests an immodest heart, religion ought to have nothing to do with those things of which virtue is ashamed to speak. Therefore, we forbid by apostolic authority this practice to continue, so that the monastic order and the order of canons may be preserved without stain in a state of life pleasing to God, in accord with their holy purpose. Furthermore, bishops, abbots and priors who consent to and fail to correct such an outrageous practice are to be deprived of their own honours and kept from the thresholds of the church.

## 5.10
## Scholastic theologies of medicine and healing
Thomas Aquinas, *Summa theologiae*[14]

*St. Thomas Aquinas (1224/25–1274) was one of the most influential Christian thinkers, at different points recognized by Roman Catholic pontiffs as a doctor of the church, a saint, a patron of Catholic schools, and a model for theologians. A Dominican friar, Aquinas spent much of his life writing, preaching, and teaching both in Italy and at the University of Paris. Known as quiet, withdrawn, and reluctant to talk in everyday interactions, Aquinas was a prolific writer who left a vast corpus of theological treatises, commentaries, and summae (ordered syntheses of Christian teachings). His (unfinished) masterpiece Summa theologiae, intended for beginners in the study of sacred doctrine, contained 512 topics and 2,668 mini-disputations and comprised more than 1.5 million words in its original form. The structure of the following excerpt was standard for the Summa's mini-disputations. A question was followed by objections, to which Aquinas responded—appealing to the Bible, philosophical works, and writings of authoritative church fathers—with both a general response and specific replies to each individual objection. This excerpt is part of the Summa's rejection on religious grounds of the employment of magical as opposed to "natural" healing methods.*

### IIaIIae. Question 96: "Superstition In Various Practices"
*Article 2: Are practices for effecting bodily changes unlawful?*

The Second Point: It would seem that practices for effecting bodily changes for the purpose of health or the like are lawful. It is legitimate to make use of the natural forces of bodies in order to produce their proper effects. Yet these have hidden powers which man is not yet capable of explaining, for instance, why a magnet attracts iron: Augustine cites many other examples (*De civitate Dei* xxi, 5,7). Therefore, it seems that to employ them for the transmutation of bodies is not unlawful.

. . .

On the Other Hand Augustine says that to superstition *belong the experiments of magic arts, amulets, and nostrums condemned by the medical faculty; they include incantations and cyphers and brooches, or any kind of charm which is worn* (*De doctrina Christiana* ii, 20).

Reply: When things are used in order to produce an effect, we have to ask whether this is produced naturally. If the answer is yes, then to use them so will not be unlawful, since we may rightly employ natural causes for their proper effects. But if they seem unable to produce the effects in question naturally, it follows that they are being used for the purpose of producing them, not as causes but only as signs, so that they come under the head of a compact entered into with the demonic. Augustine says, *demons are lured by means of creatures, which were made, not by them, but by God. They are enticed by various objects, differing according to the various things in which they delight. Not as animals by meat, but as spirits by signs, such as are to each one's liking, by means of various kinds of stones, herbs, trees, animals, songs, and rites (De civitate Dei xxi, 6).*

Hence: There is nothing superstitious or wrong in using natural things for the purpose of causing effects which are thought natural to them. But if in addition there be employed certain cyphers, words, or other vain observances, which clearly have no efficacy by nature, then this is superstitious and wrong.

## 5.11
## Medicine and witchcraft
### *Malleus Maleficarum*[15]

*Malleus Maleficarum (The Hammer of [Female] Witches) was an enormously popular late medieval guidebook for witch hunters. First published in Strasbourg in 1486–87, it was reprinted fourteen times over the next thirty-three years. While* Malleus Maleficarum *largely evoked and systematized long-existing traditional beliefs about witches, it laid out for the first time a detailed program for their persecution and legal trials, even by secular judges.*

As for the other argument, the one about how illnesses can be distinguished from each other, so that one is caused by sorcery, the other by nature, for example as a result of a defect of nature, it is answered that this can be done in various ways. The first is through the judgment of physicians (26, Q. 5, "*Non licet*" and Q. 2, "*Illud*"). In the second chapter are the words of Augustine: "To this kind of superstition belong all amulets and cures that the medical discipline condemns in connection with tying on and knotting any objects." A similar way is when physicians form, on the basis of circumstances (age, the sudden changing of a temperament that had been healthy in virtually the blinking of an eye, and the fact that the illness did not happen as the result of blood, bile or deformity), the judgment that the illness happened as the result not of a defect of nature but from an external cause. In a case where it happened from an external cause, if it did not happen as a result of tainting with poison, because in this case the blood and stomach would be filled with evil humors, then on the basis of a sufficient distinction they judge that the effect is one of sorcery. The second way is when the illness is incapable of being cured by them, so that no drugs can make the sick man better, and instead the physicians see that he is getting worse. The third way consists of the occasions when the illness happens so suddenly that the judgment of the sick man agrees about this [i.e., that it is sorcery].

## 5.12
### Physicians' sins
Antoninus Pierozzi, *Summa theologica moralis*[16]

*St. Antoninus Pierozzi (1389–1459), a Dominican archbishop of Florence, authored influential reference manuals for medieval confessors. Since a heartfelt confession of all sins was considered necessary for their absolution, it was a confessor's goal to aid penitents in fully acknowledging their transgressions. In this respect, it was useful for a confessor to be aware of the particular temptations faced by practitioners of different occupations. The following excerpt from Pierozzi's 1477 manual,* Summa theologica moralis, *describes sins commonly committed by physicians in the course of their practice.*

In the practice of their art, physicians are wont to commit offences in many ways. First, in the bodily care of the sick: here they offend from ignorance, from negligence, and sometimes from malice.

Therefore one must first look into whether the physician is expert in the art, such that he would generally be considered competent by those who are experts in this field. It is not sufficient for him to hold a doctoral degree, because these days many unworthy people are masters and doctors in every field, to their own damnation and also of those who promote them [for the degree]. Subsequently, when they harm their patients through their treatments because of conspicuous ignorance, they always commit a mortal sin. . . . Nor can they excuse themselves by claiming that they did not intend [to do harm], because they voluntarily put themselves in that position . . . and even if the outcome is healing, they are not excused from sin, because they have exposed themselves to the danger of mortal sin by an act that can result in significant harm to one's neighbor.

Secondly, a physician must exercise due diligence, for however great his expertise, if he is conspicuously negligent in consulting his books, in visiting the sick, or in [assuring] the quality of medical products, and death results, he has sinned mortally and acted irregularly. And even if the result is a considerable worsening of the illness, and not actual death, he is not excused from mortal [sin]. And therefore . . . he should exercise diligence. He is said to do this when he follows the traditions of the art, and when he visits the patient in person, and when he prescribes [the patient's] diet and regimen himself, but he is not bound to keep him under continuous personal observation, as Hostiensis says. And [the doctor] does ill by administering a medication if there is any doubt as to whether it might harm or be of benefit; for according to the dictum of Innocent [III?], in a doubtful situation, one ought rather to leave the patient in the hands of the Creator than to expose him to a medication one does not know about.

Thirdly, a physician should treat the patient as expeditiously as possible. Whence, if he deliberately omits a medication which is suitable and which would bring about a quick cure, so that [the patient] continues to be sick, in order to increase his earnings, then he sins gravely and what he has earned has been by theft. And likewise if in making up a medication he allows the apothecary to put in old spices and other things of this kind, which have no efficacy, to profit [the apothecary], when he can and ought to put in other things, he sins gravely. And if anything detrimental happens to the patient, the blame lies with both of them. In fact, a physician should not confide the compounding of medications to an apothecary, unless he knows him to have a scrupulous conscience and to be well taught and practiced in this kind of thing; rather, he should have [the medication] made up in his presence, and closely observe what goes into it.

Physicians also commit mortal sin if they give any advice or remedy for the health of the body that imperils the soul—for example, [advice] to do something against the divine law, for instance, to know a woman carnally outside matrimony, or to get drunk, or the like. . . . [I]t is a mortal sin for both the physician and the patient, for it is against the order of charity according to which the health of the soul takes precedence over that of the body. . . . And a physician who says to a patient, "I do not advise this, but were you to have sex with a woman, you would get better," transgresses this law. For when I sell you something, adding, "I do not wish to be held accountable if it is dangerous and harmful," when I know it is such, I am accountable. The physician should, therefore, beware of what he says, lest in assigning a cause to the disease he incite [the patient] to do something evil.

### 5.13
### Conciliar regulation of medical and ecclesial practices

*The Fourth Lateran Council, also known as the twelfth ecumenical council and the Great Council, took place in 1215. Summoned by Pope Innocent III, it is often regarded as the most influential medieval council prior to that of Trent. The following excerpts are from the council-approved canons 21 and 22, which address matters of spiritual and physical health.*

### *a. Canon 21*
Fourth Lateran Council[17]

All the faithful of either sex, after they have reached the age of discernment, should individually confess all their sins in a faithful manner to their own priest at least once a year, and let them take care to do what they can to perform the penance imposed on them. . . .

The priest shall be discerning and prudent, so that like a skilled doctor he may pour wine and oil over the wounds of the injured one. Let him carefully inquire about the circumstances of both the sinner and the sin, so that he may prudently discern what sort of advice he ought to give and what remedy to apply, using various means to heal the sick person.

### *b. Canon 22*
Fourth Lateran Council[18]

As sickness of the body may sometimes be the result of sin—as the Lord said to the sick man whom he had cured, *Go and sin no more, lest something worse befall you*—so we by this present decree order and strictly command physicians of the body, when they are called to the sick, to warn and persuade them first of all to call in physicians of the soul so that after their spiritual health has been seen to they may respond better to medicine for their bodies, for when the cause ceases so does the effect. This among other things has occasioned this decree, namely that some people on their sickbed, when

they are advised by physicians to arrange for the health of their souls, fall
into despair and so the more readily incur the danger of death. If any physician transgresses this our constitution, after it has been published by the
local prelates, he shall be barred from entering a church until he has made
suitable satisfaction for a transgression of this kind. Moreover, since the soul
is much more precious than the body, we forbid any physician, under pain of
anathema, to prescribe anything for the bodily health of a sick person that
may endanger his soul.

## 5.14
## Foundations of medical ethics in China
### Sun Ssu-miao, *A Thousand Golden Remedies*[19]

*Sun Ssu-miao (581–673/82 CE) was a Chinese physician and medical writer,
later recognized as a "king of medicine." He was the author of the earliest Chinese medical encyclopedia,* A Thousand Golden Remedies, *which contained
more than 5,300 medical remedies, and* Supplement to a Thousand Golden
Remedies, *which contained more than 2,000. Considered to be the founder of
Chinese medical ethics, he was likely a follower of Taoism and was also influenced by Buddhist thought. The following excerpts from his first book are a discussion of medical learning and the obligations of physicians with regard to
their colleagues and patients.*

Medicine is an art which is difficult to master. If one does not receive a divine guidance from God, he will not be able to understand the mysterious
points. A foolish fellow, after reading medical formularies for three years,
will believe that all diseases can be cured. But after practicing for another
three years, he will realize that most formulae are not effective. A physician
should, therefore, be a scholar, mastering all the medical literature and
working carefully and tirelessly. . . .

A great doctor, when treating a patient, should make himself quiet and
determined. He should not have covetous desire. He should have bowels
of mercy on the sick and pledge himself to relieve suffering among all
classes. Aristocrat or commoner, poor or rich, aged or young, beautiful or
ugly, enemy or friend, native or foreigner, and educated or uneducated, all
are to be treated equally. He should look upon the misery of the patient as
if it were his own and be anxious to relieve the distress, disregarding his

own inconveniences, such as night-call, bad weather, hunger, tiredness, etc. Even foul cases, such as ulcer, abscess, diarrhea, etc., should be treated without the slightest antipathy. One who follows this principle is a great doctor, otherwise, he is a great thief. . . .

A physician should be respectable and not talkative. It is a great mistake to boast of himself and slander other physicians. . . .

Lao Tze, the father of Taoism, said, "Open acts of kindness will be rewarded by man while secret acts of evil will be punished by God." Retribution is very definite. A physician should not utilize his profession as a means for lusting. What he does to relieve distress will be duly rewarded by Providence. . . .

He should not prescribe dear and rare drugs just because the patient is rich or of high rank, nor is it honest and just to do so for boasting.

## 5.15
## Ethics and medicine in Judaism

*Moses Maimonides (1135–1204) was a physician, religious philosopher, and scholar of Jewish religious law, whose work profoundly impacted the subsequent intellectual history of Judaism. Following the Almohad conquest, his family fled their native Spain for fear of persecution. After years of wandering, Maimonides finally settled in Old Cairo, Egypt, where he became the house physician of Saladin's vizier and a leader in the local Jewish community.*

### a. Moses Maimonides, "The Oath of Maimonides"[20]

*This excerpt is the Oath of a Physician, attributed to Maimonides. Composed in the form of a prayer, it commended learning, compassion, and the divine calling of a physician.*

The eternal providence has appointed me to watch over the life and health of Thy creatures. May the love for my art actuate me at all times; may neither avarice nor miserliness, nor thirst for glory or for a great reputation engage my mind; for the enemies of truth and philanthropy could easily deceive me and make me forgetful of my lofty aim of doing good to Thy children.

May I never see in the patient anything but a fellow creature in pain.

Grant me the strength, time and opportunity always to correct what I have acquired, always to extend its domain; for knowledge is immense and the spirit of man can extend indefinitely to enrich itself daily with new requirements.

Today he can discover his errors of yesterday and tomorrow he can obtain a new light on what he thinks himself sure of today. Oh, God, Thou has appointed me to watch over the life and death of Thy creatures; here am I ready for my vocation and now I turn unto my calling.

### b. Moses Maimonides, "On the Diseases of the Soul"[21]

*This excerpt is from the third chapter of Maimonides's* Eight Chapters on Ethics. *This work served as an introduction to his* Chapters of the Fathers *and was the third part of Maimonides's famed comprehensive study of the Talmud,* Commentary on the Mishnah, *written between 1158 and 1168. Maimonides used medical terms analogously for describing one's moral state.*

The ancients said that the soul can be healthy or sick, just as the body can be healthy or sick. The health of the soul consists in its condition and that of its parts being such that it always does good and fine things and performs noble actions. Its sickness consists in its condition and that of its parts being such that it always does bad and ugly things and performs base actions.

The health and sickness of the body are investigated by the art of medicine. Now due to the corruption of their senses, people with sick bodies imagine the sweet as bitter and the bitter as sweet. They fancy that what is suitable is not suitable; they strongly desire and take great pleasure in things that contain no pleasure at all for the healthy and which may even be painful, such as eating clay, charcoal, dirt, and things which are extremely pungent and sour, as well as similar foods which the healthy do not desire but loathe. In like manner, people with sick souls, I mean, bad and defective men, imagine bad things as good and good things as bad. The bad man always has a desire for ends that are in truth bad. Because of the sickness of his soul, he imagines them to be good.

When sick people not proficient in the art of medicine become aware of their illness, they seek out the physicians. They [the physicians] inform them of what they need to do, prohibit them from [taking] what they imagine to be pleasurable, and compel them to take vile, bitter things which will heal their bodies so that they will again delight in pleasant things and loathe vile things. Similarly, those with sick souls need to seek out the wise men, who are the physicians of the soul. The latter will prohibit the bad things which they [the sick] think are good and treat them by means of the art that treats the moral habits of the soul, as we shall explain in the next chapter.

Those with sick souls who do not recognize their illness but imagine they are healthy or who recognize it but do not submit to medical treatment will meet the fate of a sick man who pursues his pleasures and does not submit to medical treatment—he will undoubtedly perish.

## NOTES

1. One concise survey of the history of medicine in this period, accessible to a non-specialist audience, is provided by W. F. Bynum's *History of Medicine*. For a brief historical survey of Christian approaches to healing, see Porterfield's *Healing in the History of Christianity*.

2. Complex phenomena pertaining to gender, spirituality, and devotional embodied experiences of suffering in the Middle Ages are thoroughly analyzed in Caroline Walker Bynum's classic works on the subject, including *Holy Feast and Holy Fast* and *Fragmentation and Redemption*.

3. Barstow, *Witchcraze*, 23; Thurston, *Witch, Wicce, Mother Goose*, 42.

4. From *Early Christian Lives*, trans. and ed. Carolinne White (London: Penguin Classics, 1998), 203–4. Translation, notes, and introduction copyright © Carolinne White, 1998. Reproduced by permission of Penguin Books Ltd.

5. From *The Age of Bede*, trans. J. F. Webb, ed. with an introduction by D. H. Farmer (London: Penguin Classics, 1965; reprinted 1988, 1998), 74–75. Translation copyright © J. F. Webb, 1965. Introduction and notes copyright © D. H. Farmer, 1988, 1998. Reproduced by permission of Penguin Books Ltd.

6. "Life of St. Theodore of Sykeon," in Dawes, *Three Byzantine Saints*, 115–16.

7. From *The Rule of Benedict*, trans. with an introduction and notes by Carolinne White (London: Penguin Classics, 2008), 59. Editorial material and translation copyright © Carolinne White, 2008. Reproduced by permission of Penguin Books Ltd.

8. King, *The Rule, Statutes, and Customs*, 20–24.

9. Ibid., 35–40.

10. Julian of Norwich, *Showings*, 178–81.

11. Raymond of Capua, *Life of St. Catherine*, 35–36.

12. Hildegard of Bingen, *On Natural Philosophy and Medicine*, trans. Margaret Berger (Cambridge: D. S. Brewer, 1999), 39–40. Reprinted by permission of Boydell & Brewer Ltd.

13. Norman P. Tanner, *Decrees of the Ecumenical Councils* (Washington, DC: Georgetown University Press, 1990), 198–99. Copyright © 1990 by Georgetown University Press. Reprinted with permission. www.press.georgetown.edu.

14. Thomas Aquinas, *Summa theologiae*, vol. 40, ed. T. F. O'Meara and M. J. Duffy (New York: Cambridge University Press, 2006), 75–77. Reprinted with permission.

15. Christopher S. Mackay, trans., *The Hammer of Witches: A Complete Translation of the* Malleus Maleficarum (New York: Cambridge University Press, 2009), 84D, 256–57. Reprinted with permission.

16. Pierozzi, "Diverse Vices of Physicians," in *Medieval Medicine: A Reader*, ed. Faith Wallis (Toronto: University of Toronto Press, 2010), 437–38. Copyright © 2010 University of Toronto Press Incorporated. Reprinted with permission of the publisher.

17. Tanner, *Decrees of the Ecumenical Councils*, 245.

18. Ibid., 245–46.

19. T'ao Lee, "Medical Ethics in Ancient China," *Bulletin of the History of Medicine* 13.1 (1943): 268–69. Copyright © 1943 The Johns Hopkins Press. Reprinted with permission of Johns Hopkins University Press.

20. Friedenwald, "Oath and Prayer of Maimonides," n.p.

21. From Maimonides, *Ethical Writings of Maimonides*, ed. Raymond Weiss and Charles Butterworth (New York: New York University Press, 1975), 65–67. Copyright © 1975 New York University.

# SIX

# Islam

## M. A. Mujeeb Khan

## INTRODUCTION

"Islam" as a term incorporates a complex history, culture, and religion. The word's most prominent contemporary relationship is with the religion, but Islam also denotes a culture and civilization that formed and flourished as a result of this religion. The Prophet Muhammad was born in 570 CE on the Arabian Peninsula in the city of Mecca and, within little more than a century after his death in 632, Muslim rule extended from Central Asia to North Africa and the Iberian Peninsula.

When Muhammad died, an early divide developed in Islam regarding the question of whether the seat of political leadership also represented religious leadership. One side sought succession to Muhammad in the form of representative voting and a separation of these roles while the other sought for political legitimacy founded on religious authority through the family of the Prophet. This division would come to be represented by two people: the first historical successor (caliph), Abū Bakr al-Ṣiddīq (d. 634), who became a symbol for the separation between the two roles; and the fourth historical successor, a spiritual leader and son-in-law of the Prophet, ʿAlī Ibn Abī Ṭālib (d. 661), a symbol for the union of the roles. The different readings of this history led to the rise of two groups: the Shia and the Sunni. The Shia arose with a belief that placed ʿAlī as their first imam—to them, both a religious and a political leader—and his family as heirs to the prophetic legacy. In contrast, the Sunni would later be distinguished by their acceptance of the historical reality of the four successors (from Abū Bakr through ʿAlī), who ruled 632–661, as legitimate.

Following the four successors to Muhammad, Muʿawīya (d. 680) established the Umayyad dynasty (661–750 CE). Building on the expansion of territory under the earlier successors, the Umayyads achieved a further extension of their rule and a greater increase in non-Arab lands. By the eighth century, however, internal strife was prevalent in the Umayyad state. Factors including the Persianization of the Arabs and the Arabicization of the Persians, the support of the Shia, and political support from various influential groups allowed the Abbasids to overthrow the Umayyads and establish their own rule in 750 in Baghdad. The Abbasid dynasty maintained much of its political power until the sack of Baghdad in 1258 by invading Mongols from Central Asia, and it survived nominally for centuries thereafter. During this period, the Islamic world came to span what at the time was the known world of Afro-Eurasia, stretching as far as Spain and France in western Europe and Italy in southern Europe and eastward as far as Central Asia and what is now China and southeastern Asia.

The Qur'an is the central source of Islamic teachings and is said to have been revealed to the Prophet Muhammad by the angel Jibrīl (Gabriel) over a period of twenty-three years between 610 and 632. Comprising 114 suras (chapters), the Qur'an includes various types of literary genres, from stories to allegories, from prayers of praise and petition to law. Within it are many references to medicine, including the development of a spiritual tradition that imagines a spiritual body that is in parallel to its physical counterpart. The Qur'an distinguishes itself as a source of spiritual healing and identifies spiritual illnesses of the heart as a dangerous condition [6.1, 6.11]. It also addresses the physical world and healing. The complex narrative of the Qur'an makes it clear that God permits both the power of natural healing substances and the natural order of things.

In addition to the Qur'an, the teachings and actions of the Prophet serve as a basis for Islam. Collectively they are called sunna, and records of what the Prophet taught or did were transmitted as individual reports called hadith. The Qur'an and the sunna together have functioned as the basis for Islamic religious law and spirituality. Unlike the Qur'an, which was collected and collated early on, the hadith remained an oral tradition for Islam's first two centuries. From the use of black cumin seed and honey as remedies to the use of cupping as a therapy, the Prophet is reported to have recommended treatments for various ailments and illnesses. The Prophet's support of medicine is seen explicitly in his statement that "for every disease there is a remedy, and when the remedy is applied to the disease, it is cured by the permission of God" [6.2d].

The influence of the Prophet's legacy is also found in social and spiritual medicine. The former is seen in the Prophet's construction of a community [6.2e] and the latter in his imperative that Muslims improve themselves and increase their proximity to God. This requirement for self-improvement was elaborated in the works of spiritual masters in the Islamic tradition through the juxtaposition of the spiritual and the physical. In what is now called the Sufi tradition, many mystics organized their discussions of spiritual soundness in terms of states akin to their physical counterparts. Abū Ḥāmid al-Ghazālī, an exemplar of this tradition, explored various intellectual approaches to reaching God most appropriately, and he documented his journey, relating the importance of the spiritual tradition by first emphasizing the indispensability of physical medicine [6.8]. This use of physical medicine to underscore the value of the spiritual demonstrates the elevated place of medicine in the Islamic tradition. Even in the thirteenth century this medical metaphor continued to be used by spiritual masters. Ibn ʿAṭāʾ Allāh al-Iskandarī, for example, touched on this metaphor in his manual on invocation [6.10].

Interactions with the medical infrastructure of other civilizations, such as Christendom and Persia, led to a rise of hospitals in the Islamic world, which reflected the importance of public welfare. During the Umayyad dynasty hospitals first began to flourish. They utilized the waqf system, a government endowment for welfare, to provide medical care to all regardless of their ability to afford it. Under the Abbasids, the presence of hospitals became standard in several cities throughout the Islamic world.

Abū Bakr al-Rāzī's role in establishing the famous Baghdad hospital has been well recorded. Besides serving in an administrative role in hospitals, al-Rāzī was a polymath (a person of encyclopedic knowledge) and a highly influential clinician and medical writer, but he was not a participant in a religious medical tradition. In fact, his publication on spiritual medicine (*al-Ṭibb al-Rūḥānī*) was a work of normative ethics, tracing its roots to the Greek tradition of deontology.[1]

Medicine flourished in Islamic culture not only under the rubric of healing in a strictly religious sense but also in the form of a rational medical tradition largely based on the principles of Greek philosophy. Abbasid patronage and the dynasty's interest in foreign cultures led to the establishment of a translation movement. Lasting from the eighth through the tenth centuries and consisting of works from Greek, Persian, Syriac, and Sanskrit sources, the extensive Abbasid translation movement was the first of its kind. Under its auspices almost the whole corpus of secular, nonliterary, and nonhistorical Greek works available at the time was translated into Arabic. The project's international nature is evident in that the commissioned translators were speakers of Greek and Syriac, most of them neither Arab nor Muslim, but often Christian.

The importance of Islamic medicine can be seen in the recorded debates between physicians and in discussions in the works of medical writers [6.4]. The later translations into Persian, Turkish, and other languages reflected a localization and popularization of medicine that was seen in other parts of the late medieval and early modern world. Early translators of medicine—including the prominent medical translator Ḥunayn Ibn Isḥāq al-ʿIbādī (d. 873), a Nestorian Christian—provided summae (summaries) and guidebooks alongside their translations. Indian medicine also played a role in the early development of Islamic medicine, as can be seen in ʿAlī Ibn Sahl Rabbān al-Ṭabarī's (d. mid-ninth century) *Firdaws al-Ḥikma* (Paradise of Wisdom).

By the early tenth century, original rational medical writing was flourishing in the Islamic world. Following al-Rāzī, ʿAlī Ibn al-ʿAbbās al-Majūsī was an early encyclopedist. Like other early writers, al-Majūsī (known as Haly Abbas in Europe) also considered issues of medical ethics and propriety [6.5]. Medical ethics revealed the concern of writers for correctness and authority in relation to physicians and medical practices. Other prominent writers in this genre included Isḥāq Ibn ʿAlī al-Ruhāwī, who produced an extensive work on the topic [6.3] a century before al-Majūsī, and Abū al-Faraj Ibn Hindū, who outlined medicine a century later [6.6]. Similarly, ʿAbd al-Laṭīf al-Baghdādī's treatise [6.9] both critiqued physicians working for money and emphasized the nobility of the medical profession.

Medical encyclopedism was exemplified by Abū ʿAlī Ibn Sīnā, whose erudition spanned many other disciplines. Ibn Sīnā's *al-Kitāb al-qānūn fī al-Ṭibb* (Canon of Medicine) [6.7] remained for centuries an important source for medical theory and education throughout the Islamic world and in Europe, where it was widely used in its Latin translation.

Synthesizing the religious and medical literary approaches, prophetic medicine emerged in the Islamic world. As a genre, prophetic medicine drew on a specialized collection of hadith utilizing Galenic theory and included quotations from Greek and Islamic medical writers as well as Arabic folk medicine. It was prescriptive in nature and emphasized the preservation of health through a regulated life, including the maintenance of personal hygiene and moderation in diet. Prophetic medicine developed after the rise of its nonreligious counterpart and was grounded in the religious aspects of medicine drawn from the Qur'an and the sunna along with the medical literary tradition embodied in the works of al-Rāzī and Ibn Sīnā. Ibn Qayyim al-Jawzīya and al-Suyūṭī are representative of this genre, although the historicity of the latter's work has been challenged [6.11, 6.12].

In spite of the beginnings of the Islamic world, multiple empires and states came to rule over regions now associated with the contemporary Muslim world. During the late medieval and early modern periods, hospitals and medical learning were based on the rational medical tradition, drawing on the works of physicians like Ibn Sīnā. In other words, the rational medical literary tradition dominated medical education in the Islamic world in later centuries. Rational Islamic medicine moved into regions beyond the Islamic world as well. For example, Rashīd al-Dīn Faḍl Allāh Hamadānī (d. 1318) worked in the Mongol courts facilitating the translations of Chinese and Islamic cultural works. During this period, works like *Hui hui yao fang* (Islamic Formularies),[2] derived from the rational medical literary tradition, were translated into Chinese, and, similarly, Chinese works entered the Islamic world. In the West, the Islamic world engaged with a new European medicine. For example, Paracelsus's writings on chemical medicine were translated into Arabic as early as 1640. When colonial powers invaded the Islamic world, a different encounter with Europe occurred as early modern European-style medical institutions were introduced. Although Ottoman medicine flourished in the early modern period, by the late nineteenth century the disarray of medical institutions in Egypt due to neglect by the state coincided with a local negotiation of the newly encountered British medicine with already established forms of medicine in Egypt.

With the rise of modern biomedicine in the twentieth century, many of these traditions have fallen into disuse; however, both Ūnānī medicine, a preserved form of the medieval Islamic medical literary tradition focusing on the teachings of physicians such as Ibn Sīnā, and prophetic medicine continue to be popular as traditional and religious medical systems. In each of these traditions, Islam as religion and as culture plays an important role, just as it did in the imperatives of Islam's sacred texts, the writings of religious scholars, and nonreligious medical traditions.

# TEXTS

## 6.1
## From the Qur'an[3]

*The Qur'an is the source of Islamic teachings regarding both law and culture. As tradition goes, it was revealed to the Prophet Muhammad over a period of twenty-three years (610–632 CE). The later recorded teachings of the Prophet are also interpreted in the light of the Qur'an. For these reasons, the Qur'an serves as an important starting point. However, since the works on prophetic medicine excerpted later in this chapter also quote from the Qur'an, only one passage is cited here. The following quotations from chapter 16 explain the order of nature and the imperative for people to follow natural principles. This chapter also identifies the healing nature of honey.*

### Chapter 16. The bee

16.64: We have sent down the Scripture to you only to make clear to them what they differ about, and as guidance and mercy to those who believe.

16.65: It is God who sends water down from the sky and with it revives the earth when it is dead. There truly is a sign in this for people who listen.

16.66: In livestock, too, you have a lesson—We give you a drink from the contents of their bellies, between waste matter and blood, pure milk, sweet to the drinker.

16.67: From the fruits of date palms and grapes you take sweet juice {i.e., wine, vinegar, or juice} and wholesome provisions. There truly is a sign in this for people who use their reason.

16.68: And your Lord inspired the bee, saying, "Build yourselves houses in the mountains and trees and what people construct."

16.69: "Then feed on all kinds of fruit and follow the ways made easy for you by your Lord." From their bellies comes a drink of different colours in which there is healing for people. There truly is a sign in this for those who think.

## 6.2
## From the hadith

*Although they play a much less prominent role in the Shia tradition, in the Sunni tradition hadith are often given a place next to the Qur'an in Islamic discourse. The hadith therefore provide deep insight into the lived traditions of*

*Islam from its earliest teacher, the Prophet Muhammad. As with the Qur'an, the hadith figure prominently in the later tradition of prophetic medicine. The following five hadith are from the two most prominent collections: by al-Bukhārī (d. 870) and by Muslim (d. 875). They present different aspects of the way illness was seen in early Islam and the importance of seeking medical treatment.*

### a. Narrated by Abū Hurayra
Muḥammad al-Bukhārī[4]

The Prophet said, "If a house fly falls in the drink of anyone of you, he should dip it (in the drink), for one of its wings has a disease and the other has the cure for the disease."

### b. Narrated by Abū Mūsā al-Ashʿarī
Muḥammad al-Bukhārī[5]

The Prophet said, "Feed the hungry, visit the sick, and set free the captives."

### c. Narrated by Abū Hurayra
Muḥammad al-Bukhārī[6]

The Prophet said, "There is no disease that [God] has sent down except that He also has sent down its treatment."

### d. Words of the Prophet according to Jābir
Saḥīḥ Muslim[7]

"For every disease there is a remedy, and when the remedy is applied to the disease, it is cured by the permission of God."

### e. Words of the Prophet reported to have been narrated by al-Nuʿmān Ibn Bashīr
Saḥīḥ Muslim[8]

"The likeness of the believers in their mutual love, mercy and compassion is that of the body; when one part of it is in pain, the rest of the body joins it in restlessness and fever."

## 6.3
## On the physician's responsibilities
Isḥāq Ibn ʿAlī al-Ruhāwī, *Ethics of the Physician*[9]

*The earliest known text in the Arabic language on medical ethics, al-Ruhāwī's work addressed various issues related to medicine. The selection quoted here deals with the profession of medicine and physicians. Most important, while this medical text was written in Arabic in the Islamic world, the author's name hints at his Christian origins. It is uncertain whether al-Ruhāwī was Muslim or became Muslim, but his discussions are distinctly Islamic in principle.*

## On the dignity of the medical profession

Since we have mentioned the dignity of the medical art and its priority in rank to other arts and crafts, it encourages people of reason and culture to acquire it. It inspires them to desire to follow its commands and refrain from the prohibitions. It urges them to show regard for its practitioners. Therefore, it is necessary for me to mention that which is notable of its dignity, and the best of its virtues.

When I say the other arts and crafts, their complete mention is not given nor is their end attained except after imagining the science in them. Since science is of the reasonable soul and work is of the body, and since the soul is completed only by science with the body when it is healthy, and since health must be preserved, maintained, secured, and strengthened by the art of medicine, therefore, it is necessary that the art of medicine be the noblest of the arts. Its science is the oldest of the sciences. The means by which the skills and arts are developed are two; one of them is analogy, and the other is experiment.

It is not possible to extract the principles of medicine with one of them or with both together if sense does not perceive them. This comes from that which we describe. When the first one of the creatures was created in need of food, he didn't know food from a drug [since] both were from species of plants. If he took one of them blindly as food, then he took a risk and rushed headlong into peril. If he took the scammony herb, for example, or any other of the lethal herbs and ate it, he died if sense did not lead to knowledge about it. There is no way to knowledge about perceptible things and to distinguish them except through sense. Thus, it is impossible to know the principles of medical art [only] through deduction and analogy.

As to the consequence of these principles, there is no doubt as to the development of those two which I have extracted. There is no other way to obtain them unless it is in the extraordinary manner of the story of Galen. He saw someone in his dream saying to him, "Cut the vein which is in the back of your hand between the fourth and fifth fingers. You will recover from the illness you have." He had been suffering an illness whose treatment had baffled him. He cut the vein and recovered from his ailment. We say that we do not deny those matters influenced by prophecy and soothsaying but we say that it is also because of its nobility. It is through this kind of teaching that the principles of the medical art have been learned. Galen described this in his commentary on the books of the Testaments of Hippocrates and his belief. We say that the medical art is a teaching of the exalted God, and a gift and kindness to mankind. For this reason, we have previously mentioned some of what he said on this occasion at the beginning of our book. Thus, we do not have to repeat here what was said there.

If the matter is as we have stated, then the medical art is a divine one. He who has acquired it travels a godly road and deserves this noble name if he is ambitious and does his best to imitate the acts of the exalted Creator. This is because it is enough to know that the Creator is generous, kind, merciful, sympathetic, and health-giving to the healthy. He maintains their health for them and makes the ill recover from their ailments. Truly, He is able to maintain health perfectly and cure the ill.

It is known that the intention of the physician is to request one's health and his aim is to obtain it. He cannot do this except by the art of medicine whose intention and aim is this [of requesting health and securing it]. It is given as a gift by the exalted God.

. . .

This makes clear that the medical art has nobility and that it bears many benefits for all the people. The first value which occurs to the understanding one is the acknowledgment of the oneness of the Creator, to know his fine wisdom, his great power, the beauty of his kindness to creatures at the time of contemplation of the mixing of many mixtures, the compounding compositions as solid objects with all their differences and plants in the abundance of their species and different species of animals, and then the exclusive attribution to each species especially mankind. When a man wishes to know himself and to study his complexion and organs and their forms, measures, positions, divisions, values, activities, and benefits, etc., then he will know certainly that for all these things there is one able, wise Creator who fashioned all creatures in the best form, most secure, most beautiful, and most fit. The wise man sees the result of this fruit [i.e., the body] and profits by it.

It possesses another value for it is the greatest assistant to fulfill divine law since it is possible for men to acquire science and to fulfill religious duty as fasting and prayer, etc., only when the body is healthy. To him, science is in two parts; science of the body, and science of religion. The dignity of medicine precedes the science of religion in benefit. The art of medicine is very great in dignity and profit.

There is a third value. It is for the one who seeks it for its sake, for the benefit of the people. It is not to earn money but it helps him to acquire a continuous pleasure, useful wealth, fame, and numerous divine rewards. It helps to attain dignity which brings you near God, contents, and helps attain benefits. You see then that the art of medicine is acknowledged and its dignity is from the wise men? The people of the various professions agree to its truth and its profit.

. . .

It is like what Galen did, in the superiority of his art, when he foretold what would happen. They wondered at his judgment and said that this was not by the art of medicine but, perhaps, by a kind of prophecy. This is like the story of a maiden in love whose case was diagnosed when he [Galen] felt her pulse. There are many [stories] like this in a separate treatise by him whose title is "Tales of the Introduction of Knowledge." He who wants to learn all of these may do so from this treatise. All of these cannot be done except by the power of this art. Thus it deserves nobility and priority over the other arts. Don't you see the obedience of the people of the country to their king, and the obedience of the king to his physician more than to his parents, his court, and his people? He discloses secrets to him that he will not reveal to them so that the benefit and advantage be with him.

It is told of Jibrīl, the physician of al-Ma'mūn, that he once said to him, "O Commander of the Believers, I have improved the brains of kings and cadis for fifty years, so how can I be compared with another, and confidence displayed in him!" Further, the confidants of kings and similar people disclose secrets to their physician. These are secrets which should not be revealed to their men. Thus, the dignity of medicine and the priority of its practitioners are more necessary than are men of other arts and crafts.

Perhaps, someone will say that the philosophy which rectifies the soul is more worthy of dignity than the medical art. We can answer that philosophy, indeed, is noble because of the dignity of its subject. However, you cannot consider it as medicine for the soul for then every philosopher would be a physician, and every physician who is virtuous would be a philosopher physician. The philosopher can only improve the soul, but the virtuous physician can improve both body and soul. The physician deserves the assertion that he is imitating the acts of God, the Exalted, as much as he can. This is part of the definition of philosophy. What we have mentioned in this chapter is sufficient.

**6.4**
**Shortcomings of earlier writers**
Abū Bakr Zakarīyā al-Rāzī, "On the Benefits of Nutrition
and Dispelling Its Harms"[10]

*Acknowledged to be one of the most innovative and successful clinicians, al-Rāzī (Latin, Rhazes, d. 925/932) was a prolific writer whose expertise spanned many fields. He is most famous for his medical works, especially his larger encyclopedia,* Kitāb al-Ḥāwī fī al-Ṭibb *(Latin, Liber Continens), and shorter,* Kitāb al-Manṣūrī fī al-Ṭibb *(Latin, Liber Medicinalis ad Almansorem), which circulated popularly throughout Europe. The passage quoted here, which has been translated into English for this volume, describes al-Rāzī's approach to medicine and his reason for writing texts, in particular his use of works originally from the Greek tradition and those written in the Islamic tradition.*

I decided to write a book on dispelling completely the harm of nutrition, investigating {what} I clarify and explain from the work of the eminent Galen. For he has neglected much and erred repeatedly in his book. In this sense, few have examined this, especially Yaḥyā Ibn Masawayh, for the book he produced on this matter is more harmful than beneficial, and I have a dislike for mentioning the deficiencies and reasons to which the natural philosophers are devoted. . . . From here we begin by saying that people, in their diet, depend on bread, water, drink, and meat, and, as many among them were using things other than these, I have decided to begin with a discussion of it.

## 6.5
## Ethical directives for the practice of medicine
'Alī Ibn al-'Abbās al-Majūsī, "Complete Book on the Art of Medicine"[11]

*The brilliance of Al-Majūsī (Latin, Haly Abbas, d. 994) is seen in the organization and logic of his* Kitāb Kāmil al-Ṣinā'a fī al-Ṭibb *(Complete Book on the Art of Medicine). In his text, al-Majūsī provided a straightforward and easy-to-understand outline of medicine. If not for Ibn Sīnā (Avicenna), al-Majūsī's work would have had more prominence in the world of medicine. The passage selected here, which has been translated into English for this volume, is on medical ethics and the rules a physician must follow.*

### On the advice of Hippocrates and others from the ancient scholar-physicians, by which a physician should model himself

I state that the one who desires to be a wise, scholarly physician should follow the advice of Hippocrates, which he instructed in his oath to scholar-physicians after him. {After the worshiping of God and the obeying of his commands,} I state that, first, these {people} are advised to be graciously disposed to their teachers and endeavor to hold them in esteem, to serve and show gratitude to them, to show them great piety as children show to their parents, and to share with them their possessions. Take notice of what he {Hippocrates} said, "For, as parents are the reason for one's existence, one's teachers are the cause for one's distinction, renown, and excellence in terms of knowledge; for this reason, a teacher has a right over a person just as his parents do."

. . .

Prohibit those who are undeserving, the lowly and wicked, from studying medicine. I exhort physicians to treat the sick and take good care of them through nutrition and drugs, but they should not treat them in order to achieve monetary objectives except for compensation and payment. Physicians should not prescribe any harmful drugs.

. . .

He {Hippocrates} also stated that a physician should be chaste, pure, religious, pious, well-spoken, and graceful. He should avoid sinfulness and impurity. He should not look upon women with lust nor should he go to their homes except when visiting the sick. A physician should respect privacy and protect the patient's secrets. In protecting a patient's privacy, {the physician} must be more vigilant than the patient. A physician should follow what Hippocrates has stated. He must be kind, compassionate, merciful, and benevolent and should provide treatment generously to patients, especially the poor. He must never expect remuneration from the poor but rather provide drugs for free. If it is possible, he should visit patients whenever needed, day or night, especially when they suffer from acute diseases, because the condition of a patient with such a disease worsens very quickly.

A physician should not live luxuriously and engage in hedonist activities. He should not drink alcohol because it harms the brain. . . . He should preoccupy himself with medical books every day and not desist from their study. It is necessary for him to memorize what he has read . . . and memorize what is needed from it for the science and practice {of medicine}. . . . He should conduct this memorization in his youth because it is easier to master the subject at this age than in old age. A student of this art must be in the hospital in order to see the symptoms of the sick and disease complications while around learned and proficient physicians.

. . .

It is necessary for one who desires to be a learned physician to follow this advice and develop one's character as we have noted here without hesitating to put it into practice, for this is an effective treatment for patients and this will earn the people's trust.

## 6.6
## On the medical profession
Abū al-Faraj ʿAlī Ibn al-Ḥusayn Ibn Hindū, *The Key to Medicine and a Guide for Students*[12]

*As with many early writers, the origins of Ibn Hindū (d. 1032) are unknown, and he has been identified as an Indian, a Persian, and even an Arab. Ibn Hindū largely worked in Persia as a practicing physician. The following is a fairly long excerpt from his work on medicine for physicians and students. This passage demonstrates how Ibn Hindū and people of this period in the Islamic world understood medical practice, including medicine as a discipline. It also provides contemporary perspectives on the medical profession, a profession that Ibn Hindū attempted to defend.*

## Chapter 2. On the importance of the profession of medicine

Specialists in the rational sciences do not disagree over the importance of medicine, nor do they refrain from giving it preference and from recognizing its prestige. Similar views are held by ordinary people who possess sound minds and keen insight. As for those who only claim to have knowledge of the sciences, and the common people stamped with the qualities of ignorance, they will sometimes deny the value of medicine and tend to ignore it and to persuade others to disclaim it.

Some of those who deny the existence of medicine do so to bolster up their tendency for idleness, being envious of anyone with a profession. Others do so in the false belief that the ability of a man to cure diseases and to allay suffering is an infringement of the will of God, the Exalted, and a contradiction of His wishes with regard to mankind.

. . .

Scholars proceeded to observe coincidences and to deduce distinctive characteristics on the basis of their experience. They compared their findings with basics already established through observation and by seeing with the naked eye. It is through this process that the medical profession developed in India, Persia and Byzantium; people there made use of their knowledge and advanced well beyond ignorant nations that depended on nature to cure their bodies, such as the [Bedouin] Arabs, the Turks, the Slavs and the Zanj.

It is for this reason that Hippocrates wrote in the opening to his book entitled *The Aphorisms*: "Life is short, the art is long, and time is fleeting."

In explanation of this, it is said that Hippocrates encouraged writing books on medicine, and drew attention to those who did so. If the life of one person is too short to master the profession of medicine, then it is essential to record what each man has discovered so that the profession will be complete through the efforts of many.

Here, we must speak about those who deny the existence of the medical profession. With regard to idlers, it is no more our task than that of other professions to argue with them, for they are happy with their laziness and tend to deny all crafts.

I believe these belong to the people that Aristotle forbade arguing with and, instead, instructed that prayers should be said for their salvation, or that they should be educated and properly trained.

In *The Book of Dialectics*, [Aristotle] says that there should be no debate on certain matters / because of their obscurity and subtleness, and because such matters require deep thought and deliberation; they do not get resolved by hurried thought or borrowed statements. Examples are the question of "the part" [particle] and the issue of whether [the world] is eternal or created.

. . .

Observe—may God fortify you—those who deny medicine. You will find that they are blind to the brightness of the Sun and that they deny the break of dawn. They persist in their denial of medicine even though people, high and low, are witness to the benefit they get from doctors and to the successful results of most treatment.

Observe also how the denigrator of the medical profession defies public policy by depriving people of its benefit and by preventing them from enjoying the comforts of life. Can there be anyone more in need of being granted [sound] feeling, or of being reprimanded as a criminal? From God we seek help.

With regard to those who fear that medicine is an infringement of the will of God, the Almighty and / Exalted, is it their duty then to refrain from eating when hungry and from drinking when thirsty? Perhaps God had ordained that they should perish from hunger and thirst and that, by eating or drinking, they would be going against his wishes and fulfilling their own!

If you were to look closely at any therapy—may God protect you—you will find that it is like eating when hungry and drinking when thirsty. A person who is feverish is given a cool drink by his doctor and a person who feels cold is given something to give him warmth, while one who has constipation is given a laxative and one who has diarrhoea is given a constipating remedy. Lay people's knowledge of medicine is made up of fragments and of scattered bits of contradictory information, while a physician's knowledge is a well-knit whole combining distinct parts.

It should come as no surprise that my answer to those who deny the existence of medicine should be to abstain from food and drink when hungry and thirsty, for their beliefs will lead them to undertake even graver action.

. . .

Professions can therefore be divided into two categories:

One whose existence—from beginning to end—is dependent on man, such as carpentry and goldsmithing.

The other includes skills whose beginnings are related to man, but whose completion is dependent on God, the Almighty and Exalted, and on nature, an example being farming. The tasks of tilling the soil, sowing the seeds, and irrigating the land depend on the farmer, but the growth and health of the plants are in the hands of God, the Exalted.

Medicine is of the latter category, for God, the Almighty and Exalted, designed the human body to be a guardian of its own health. Should health suffer and the guardian be able to deal with the malady through nutrition or medicine, the danger would be lifted and good health restored.

This "guardian" is known by physicians as "nature," and by legal scholars as "guardian angel." Hippocrates was referring to it when he said, "Nature is sufficient for curing diseases."

The physician is a servant of nature and has no part to play in healing, apart from providing nature with the tools needed to preserve health and to keep away disease. As for regaining health, that depends on a number of factors: nature's strength, the amenability of the body to that influence, the suitability of the tools to the task, and the absence of impediments between nature and the intended aim.

### 6.7
### On the definition of medicine
Abū ʿAlī Ibn Sīnā, "Canon of Medicine"[13]

*A self-proclaimed autodidact, Ibn Sīnā (Latin, Avicenna, d. 1035) was even more prolific a writer than al-Rāzī. In addition, while al-Rāzī was disparaged for his work on philosophy, Ibn Sīnā's peripatetic philosophy gained such popularity that it influenced later Islamic and European philosophy. His medical works were also influential. His Canon of Medicine was used in European universities through the early modern period and continues to be a source of Ūnānī medicine in South Asia. Below is a selection that has been translated for this volume from that work, which was completed during Ibn Sīnā's travels through Central Asia, as noted by his most famous student, al-Jūzjānī.*

I say that medicine is the discipline that discloses the states of the body as to what is a state of health and what removes one from a state of health, in order to preserve one's health when acquired and restore it when lost.

. . .

And what we mean by practice is neither practice by action nor the use of bodily movement, but {what we mean} is a branch of medical knowledge that facilitates the formation of an opinion, and that opinion pertains to how to practice {i.e., what to do}.

## 6.8
## On teaching and medicine
### Abū Ḥāmid al-Ghazālī, *Path to Sufism and His Deliverance from Error*[14]

*Al-Ghazālī (Latin, Algazel, d. 1111), erroneously thought to have closed the Islamic world to rational and foreign learning, was a jurist and Sufi mystic. Before leaving for seclusion, al-Ghazālī had become a well-known teacher, having studied philosophy, jurisprudence, and theology. Upon his return he became one of the most famous scholars in Islamic history through his Iḥyā' 'Ulūm al-Dīn (Revival of the Religious Sciences). In his autobiography, he detailed his path to Sufism and recounted his return to teaching because of society's need for doctors of the heart.*

### Reason for resuming teaching after having given it up
*A. Doctor of hearts*

For nearly ten years I assiduously cultivated seclusion and solitude. During that time several points became clear to me of necessity for reasons I cannot enumerate—at one time by fruitional experience, at another time by knowledge based on apodeictic proof, and again by acceptance founded on faith. These points were: that man is formed of a body and a heart—and by the "heart" I mean the essence of man's spirit which is the seat of the knowledge of God, not the flesh which man has in common with corpse and beast; that his body may have a health which will result in its happiness, and a malady in which lies its ruin; that his heart, likewise, may have a health and soundness—and only he will be saved "who comes to God with a sound heart" (26.89), and it may have a malady which will lead to his everlasting perdition in the next life, as God Most High has said: "In their hearts is a malady" (2.9/10); that ignorance of God is the heart's deadly poison, disobedience to God its incapacitating malady, knowledge of God Most High its quickening antidote, and obedience to Him by resisting passion its healing remedy; that the only way to treat the heart by removing its malady and regaining its health lies in the use of remedies, just as that is the only way to treat the body.

Remedies for the body effectively procure health because of a property in them which men endowed with intellect cannot perceive by virtue of their intellectual resources, but rather it must be the object of blind obedience to the physicians who learned it from the prophets, who, because of the special attribute of prophecy, came to know the special properties of things. In a similar fashion it became necessarily evident to me that the reason for the effectiveness of the remedies of the acts of worship, with their prescriptions and determined quantities ordained by the prophets, cannot be perceived by means of the intellectual resources of men endowed with intellect. On the contrary, they must be the object of blind obedience to the prophets who perceived those qualities by the light of prophecy, not by intellectual resources.

Moreover, just as medicaments are composed of mixtures of elements differing in kind and quantity, some of them being double others in weight and quantity, and just as the difference of their quantities is not without a profound significance pertaining to the kind of the properties, so, likewise, the acts of worship, which are the remedies of hearts, are composed of actions differing in kind and quantity, so that a prostration is the double of a bowing, and the morning prayer is half as long as the afternoon prayer. This difference is not without a profound significance which pertains to the kind of the properties knowable only by the light of the prophecy. Very stupid and ignorant would be the man who would wish to discover in them a wisdom by means of reason, or who would suppose that they had been mentioned by chance, and not because of a profound divine significance in them which requires them to be such because of the special property in them. And just as in medicaments there are basic elements which are their chief ingredients and additional substances which are their complements, each of them having a special effect on the workings of their basic elements, so, likewise, supererogatory prayers and customary practices are complements for perfecting the effects of the principal elements of the acts of worship.

In general, then, the prophets (Peace be upon them!) are the physicians for treating the maladies of hearts. By its activity reason is useful simply to acquaint use with this fact, to bear witness to prophecy by giving assent to its reality, to certify its own blindness to perceiving what the "eye" of prophecy perceives, and to take us by our hands and turn us over to the prophets as blind men are handed over to guides and as troubled sick men are handed over to sympathetic physicians. To this point reason can proceed and advance, but it is far removed from anything beyond that except for understanding what the physician prescribes. These, then, are the insights we gained with a necessity analogous to direct vision during the period of our solitude and seclusion.

## 6.9
### Religious aspects of medicine
'Abd al-Laṭīf Ibn Yūsuf al-Baghdādī,
*The Book of the Two Pieces of Advice*[15]

*'Abd al-Laṭīf Ibn Yūsuf al-Baghdādī (d. 1231) was an important post-Ghazālī figure. Al-Ghazālī's alleged condemnation of nonreligious learning purportedly closed the doors to earlier flourishing disciplines. However, al-Baghdādī's narrative below provides evidence of how the art of medicine was seen in the thirteenth century. Written from the perspective of rational medicine, this work also sheds light on the religious imperative and importance of medicine.*

But we will commence by stating that the art of medicine is an honorable and respectable art, the merits of which are acknowledged by the general public. The people set aside their differences, made a covenant and came together to legitimate the art of medicine, so that the need for it became greater. In the art of medicine we are able to find revelation, divine inspiration, and authentic visions which were attributed to the prophets, peace be upon them, and the divine sages. The art of medicine was brought about during sleep by those who were closest to God, may he be praised and glorified. The one who made an effort in the art of medicine was not denied his (high) rank of glory and his praise was not withheld from him by all (other) parties. Verily, (all of) this reveals the merits, benefits and deeds of the art of medicine, which resembles magic.

However, those (spongers), who asked, or demanded *rizq* [subsistence, i.e., just to make profits and gains] (without having earned it, or giving something in return) extinguished the light of the art of medicine, made its memory vanish, obliterated its merits, slandered its good reputation, lowered its rank, and caused it to fail and have shortcomings. When the conditions [*shurūṭ*] of the medical art are fully adhered to, then it never makes a mistake. The skillful physician only errs occasionally, but gets things right a hundred times, as Galen said. Moreover, his miss will be neither small [decisive], nor great nor far removed from a hit [from what is correct].

## 6.10
### Remembrance and physical health
Ibn ʿAṭāʾ Allāh al-Iskandarī, *The Key to Salvation*[16]

*Ibn ʿAṭāʾ Allāh (d. 1309) is best known for his* al-Ḥikam al-ʿAṭāʾīya *(The Aphorisms of Ibn ʿAṭāʾ Allah). The* Ḥikam *has been commented on by various spiritual masters throughout history, including contemporary scholars. Ibn ʿAṭāʾ
Allāh, a Sufi mystic, was one of the most recognized members of the Shādhilī
order. Besides the* Ḥikam, *he was known for writing a systematic meditation
manual called* The Key to Salvation *(Miftāḥ al-Falāḥ). In the excerpt below
he discusses principles of the body in terms of medical principles.*

### Introduction: On the nature of remembrance
### and its explanation
#### *Section [2]*

Remembrance is like a fire that neither stays nor spreads. When it enters a
house, it says, "It is I; there is no one else but Me," which is one of the meanings of "There is no divinity but God." If it finds kindling inside, it con-
sumes it and becomes fire. If it finds darkness therein, it becomes light, thus
illuminating the house. If there is already a light in the house, then it becomes "light upon light."

Likewise with the body: invoking removes from it impure substances
which are due to intemperance in eating or result from consuming forbidden
foods. As for what is obtained from lawful food, it does not affect it. When
the injurious parts are burned away and the sound parts remain, every part
will be heard invoking as if the trumpet had been blown.

## 6.11
### Religion and medicine I
Ibn Qayyim al-Jawzīya, *Medicine of the Prophet*[17]

*Ibn Qayyim al-Jawzīya (d. 1350) was a famous polymath of the fourteenth
century and a student of Ibn Taymīya. Ibn Qayyim was trained in multiple
arts, and many of his writings survive. The selections below from his work on*

*prophetic medicine identify three important characteristics of medicine: its importance as an art, the relationship between the art and religion (i.e., Islam), and aspects of treatment. The passages also identify features of Islamic spirituality and the importance of spiritual medicine in prophetic medicine.*

## Chapter 1. Introduction and general considerations

*Praise be to God, the Lord of the Worlds, and His blessings on the noblest of Messengers, Muḥammad, Seal of the Prophets, and his family and Companions, on them all.*

These are some useful chapters on the guidance of the Prophet {peace be upon him} concerning the medicine which he used, was treated with, or recommended for others. We shall elucidate what it contains of wisdom which is not accessible to the intellects of the greatest physicians.

We ask help from God, and from Him we draw strength and power.

### a. The two types of sickness

We begin by declaring that sickness is of two kinds: sickness of the heart, and sickness of the body, both mentioned in the Qur'ān.

Sickness of the heart is of two kinds: Sickness of uncertainty and doubt, and sickness of desire and temptation, and these both appear in the Qur'ān. Concerning sickness of uncertainty, the Most High has said: "In their hearts is a disease; and God has increased their disease" (2:10). Again, He said:

"That those in whose hearts is a disease, and the unbelievers, may say: What does God mean by this as a parable?" (74:31).

### b. Principles of bodily illness

On bodily sickness, He has spoken: "There is no blame upon the blind, nor one born lame, nor on the one who is sick . . ." (24:61). He mentioned bodily sickness in connection with pilgrimage, fasting and ablution, for an amazing reason that indicates the glory of the Qur'ān, and how sufficient it is for the one who truly comprehends it. The rules of bodily medicine are three: preservation of health, expulsion of harmful substances, and protection from harm. Thus the Most High has mentioned these three principles in these three most relevant places: In the verse on fasting He said: "If any of you is ill, or on a journey, (then fasting should be made up from) a set number of other days" (2:184). For He permitted a sick person to break the fast because of illness; and the traveller in order to preserve his health and strength, as fasting while travelling might cause injury to health through the combination of vigorous movement and the consumption of the vital bodily energy which often is not properly replaced due to lack of food. So He permitted the traveller to break his fast.

. . .

In the verse of ablution the Most High referred to the protection from harm: "If you are sick, or on a journey, or one of you comes from the privy, or you have been in contact with women, and you can find no water, then take for yourselves clean sand or earth" (4:43). He permitted the sick person to desist from using water and to use earth instead, in order to protect the body against harm. There again the attention is drawn to take the necessary precautionary measures against anything which could harm the body, internally or externally.

The Most High has thus guided His servants to the three main principles of medicine and the total sum of its numerous rules. We shall mention the guidance of the Messenger of God concerning these, and shall elucidate how his guidance is the most perfect.

### c. Medicine of the heart

As for Medicine of the Heart, this has been entrusted to the Messengers, God's blessings and peace upon them; there is no means of obtaining this, except through their teaching and at their hands. For the tranquility of the heart is obtained through recognition of its Lord and Creator, His Names and Attributes, His actions and judgements; and it should prefer what He approves of and loves, and should avoid what He forbids and dislikes. Only thus can true health and life be found, and there is no path to acquire these save through the Messengers. Any idea that health of the heart can be achieved except by following them is an error on the part of the one who so thinks unless he only means the life and health of his animal soul and its desires, while the life of his heart, its health and strength, are totally ignored. If anyone does not distinguish between the one and the other, he should weep over the life of this heart, as it should be counted among the dead, and over its light, for it is submerged in the seas of darkness.

### d. Medicine of the body

Medicine of the body is of two kinds:

1. The first kind is in accordance with God's creation of the animals, both rational beings and dumb animals, and it does not require the intervention

of a physician. Treatment of hunger and thirst, cold, weariness, and suchlike is by their opposites and by that which will put an end to these states.

2. The second kind is that which requires thought and reflection: such as repelling "similar" illnesses, occurring in the temperament, thus unbalancing the equilibrium, whether erring towards heat or cold, dryness or moisture, or a combination of two of these. This is itself of two kinds: either material or qualitative, that is, either through the secretion of a matter, or the appearance of a condition. The difference between them is that illness of condition appears when the matters which actually caused it have ceased to exist, for while these matters abate, their effects remain as a condition within the temperament. But illnesses of matter are reinforced by their own causes; and when the cause of an illness remains along with it, then one must first pay attention to the cause, secondly to the illness itself, and thirdly to the medicine for it.

### e. Religion and medicine

Where does the medical knowledge of the physicians stand in relation to the Revelation which God revealed to His Messenger as to what would benefit or harm him? The relationship of the physicians' medicine to this Revelation is similar to the relationship of their sciences to what the prophets taught. Religious and prophetic medicines heal certain illnesses that even the minds of great physicians cannot grasp, and which their science, experiments and analogical deductions cannot reach. Such are the medicines of heart and soul, which promote the strength of the heart and its reliance upon God; its complete trust in Him, and taking refuge with Him; dejectedness and submission in His presence; humility towards Him; almsgiving and supplication, repentance and seeking forgiveness; beneficence towards humankind, and giving succour to the troubled and relief to the distressed. All humanity has tested these remedies, and despite their differences of creed and religion, they have found them to have a great influence in healing such as cannot be attained by the medicine of the most learned of physicians, nor by their experiments or deductions.

### *Chapter 2. Natural and divine treatment*

Treatment of illness by the Prophet {peace be upon him} was of three types: (1) with natural medicines; (2) with divine medicines; and (3) with a combination of the two. We shall speak of the three types of his guidance, beginning with the natural medicines which he prescribed and used, then the divine medicines, then the combined.

We shall merely give an indication of all this, for the Messenger of God {peace be upon him} was sent as a guide to call people to God and His Paradise, and to give knowledge of God, making clear to the Community what pleases Him and commanding them accordingly, and what angers Him and forbidding them accordingly; to teach them about the prophets and messengers, and their lives within their respective communities, and about the creation of the world, about the beginning and the end, and that which causes suffering or happiness for mankind.

As for the guidance of the Prophet {peace be upon him} on physical medicine, it came as a completion of his religious law (*sharī'a*) and equally to be used when needed. When it is not needed, one's concern and energy should be directed to the treatment of heart and soul, the preservation of health, treating illnesses, and protection against harm. That is its first purpose. Restoration of the body without restoration of the heart is of no benefit, whereas damage to the body while the spirit is restored brings limited harm, for it is a temporary damage which will be followed by a permanent and complete cure. And from God comes success.

## 6.12
## Religion and medicine II
'Abd al-Raḥmān Jalāl al-Dīn al-Suyūṭī, *As-Suyuti's* Tibb an-Nabbi[18]

*Like Ibn Qayyim al-Jawzīya, al-Suyūṭī (d. 1505) was a prolific scholar of various Islamic sciences. He authored a work on the medicine of the Prophet, in which he cited Ibn Qayyim and other earlier writers. The selection below identifies two important aspects of medicine: the state of the body and approaches to treatment. Although al-Suyūṭī's work was composed eight centuries after the rise of Islam, it showed the continued importance of medicine in the religious tradition of Islam.*

### The states of the body

Now, health is a physical condition in which all the functions are healthy. Being restored to good health is the best gift of Allah to man. It is impossible to act rightly and to pay proper attention to the obedience which is due to our Lord except when health is present. There is nothing like it. Let the worshipper give thanks for his health and never be ungrateful.

The Prophet said, may Allah bless him and grant him peace, "There are two gifts of which many men are cheated—good health and leisure." Al-Bukhari transmitted this *ḥadīth*.

The Prophet said, may Allah bless him and grant him peace, "There are worshippers of Allah whom He protects from death in battle and from sickness. He makes them live in good health and die in good health, and yet He grants them the stations of His martyrs."

Abu'd-Darda said, "O Prophet, if I am cured of my sickness and am thankful for it, is it better than if I were sick and bore it patiently?" And the Prophet, may Allah bless him and grant him peace, replied, "Truly the Prophet loves good health, just as you do."

## Principles of treatment

Whoever is given the right to practice the treatment of disease must pay attention to age, habit, function and occupation in his treatment.

. . .

Hippocrates said, "May the physician be given strength from God the Almighty, and obedience towards Him, and good advice, and an understanding of the secrets of disease. Truly he must not administer any fatal drug, nor indicate it, nor point it out. He must not give anything to a woman to cause an abortion. He must keep well away from all pollution and defilement. He must not gaze at women. He must not go in search of excess, idling away his time in pleasure, sleep, eating and drinking, or play—but he must be eager to treat the poor and the people who have nothing. He must be gentle in his speech, kind with his words, and near to God."

This is what Hippocrates said, and he was not one of the believers. I have already said that this Hippocrates was the founder of the Art of Medicine and its leader. He was a Greek physician and their father. He is regarded as having been perfect in the Art of Medicine. It is said that the tomb of Hippocrates is still visited to this day.

### NOTES

1. This work was translated by Arthur J. Arberry as *The Spiritual Physick of Rhazes* (London: John Murray, 1950).

2. This work does not survive except for the table of contents of the second half and three chapters of at least thirty.

3. M. A. S. Abdel Haleem, trans., *The Qur'an* (Oxford: Oxford University Press, 2004), 170. Oxford World's Classics. By permission of Oxford University Press.

4. Book 59, hadith 3320, in al-Bukhārī, *Translation of the Meanings of Sahîh Bukhârî*, 4:322.

5. Book 75, hadith 5649, ibid., 7:310.

6. Book 76, hadith 5678, ibid., 7:326.

7. Book 39, hadith 5741, in al-Hajjāj, *English Translation of Sahih Muslim*, 6:55.

8. Book 45, hadith 6586, ibid., 6:450–51.

9. Al-Ruhāwī, *Ethics of the Physician*, ch. 12, "On the Dignity of the Human Person," trans. Martin Levey, in Martin Levey, "Medical Ethics of Medieval Islam with Special Reference to al-Ruhāwī's 'Practical Ethics of the Physician,'" *Transactions of the American Philosophical Society* 57.3 (1967): 70–71 (Philadelphia: American Philosophical Society, 1967). Reprinted with permission.

10. al-Rāzī, *Kitāb Manāfiʿ al-Aghdhiya wa Dafʿ*, 2.

11. Al-Majūsī, *Kitāb Kāmil al-Ṣināʿa fī al-Ṭibb*, 21r–v.

12. Ibn Hindū, *Ibn al-Hindu: The Key to Medicine and a Guide for Students*, ch. 1, "On Encouraging the Study of Professions in General and the Profession of Medicine in Particular," 3–13.

13. Ibn Sīnā, *al-Kitāb al-Qānūn fī al-Ṭibb*, 13.

14. Al-Ghazālī, *Al-Ghazali's Path to Sufism*, 64–66.

15. From N. Peter Joosse, trans., *The Physician as a Rebellious Intellectual* (Frankfurt: Peter Lang, 2014), 65–66. Reprinted with permission. www.peterlang.com.

16. Ibn ʿAṭāʾ Allāh al-Iskandarī, *The Key to Salvation: A Sufi Manual of Invocation*, trans. Mary Ann Koury Danner (Cambridge: Islamic Texts Society, 1996), 48. Reprinted with permission.

17. Ibn Qayyim al-Jawzīya, *Medicine of the Prophet*, trans. Penelope Johnstone (Cambridge: Islamic Texts Society, 1998), 3–9, 17. Reprinted with permission.

18. al-Suyūṭī, *As-Suyuti's* Tibb an-Nabbi: *Medicine of the Prophet*, ed. Ahmad Thomson, adapted from a translation by Cyril Elgood (London: Ta-Ha Publishers, 2015), 6–7, 28–29. Reprinted with permission.

# SEVEN

# The Early Modern Period

## INTRODUCTION

In this chapter I explore the development of the relationship between medicine and religion in the early modern era, with particular attention to Christianity. The main focus of the chapter is the Protestant and Catholic Reformations in sixteenth-century Europe, a critical period for the subsequent global history of Christianity and the multiplicity of ways in which it came to interact with medicine. The texts I have selected highlight competing Christian interpretations, probing questions, and moral guidelines regarding medicine, diseases, and healing in that era. I further trace some of the themes of religious engagement with medicine that arose during the medieval period (discussed in chapter 5) and note the (re)emergence of distinct early modern concerns.

The early modern period is conventionally defined as stretching roughly from the fall of Constantinople to the Ottoman army (1453) through the twilight of the age of Enlightenment and the beginning of the French Revolution (1789). This historic period has special significance for the history of Christianity as a world religion. It included the emergence of Protestantism, which eventually became a third global form of the Christian religion. It saw Roman Catholic reforms, which defined and strengthened the boundaries of distinctly Catholic teachings and practices. Orthodox Christianity in the East suffered permanent losses owing to the political expansion of the Islamic Ottoman Empire, while gains were made by both Catholicism and Protestantism in the New World. It was also a period of important milestones in the history of medicine, with empirically based methods of obtaining anatomical knowledge gradually superseding medieval "library medicine" as modern scientific medicine was emerging.

With regard to the relationship between medicine and religion, early modern thinkers displayed continuity with previous epochs in exploring answers to inherited questions in changing contexts and also posed novel questions. As an age of reform in both medicine and religion, the early modern era increasingly witnessed the extensive critical probing of ideas and practices pertaining to Christianity and healing transmitted from the Middle Ages. This frequently resulted in the abandonment of those ideas and practices or their transformation in response to new realities. Protestants were not the first to question certain expressions of medieval bodily asceticism, the pursuit of saints' intercession for attaining bodily cures, and the common acceptance of a widespread ongoing reality of miraculous healings. But the critique of such staples of medieval Catholic religion gained a special force in the early Reformation and became a distinct mark of Protestant teachings. At the same time, emergent Protestantism generated renewed debates about the relationship between the spiritual and the material, resulting in the production of new models of theologically accounting for, affirming, or marginalizing medical practices. Yet a number of the older understandings of normative engagements of Christianity with medicine—albeit in changing contexts—persisted into the early modern era across confessional divides. These included a perceived ethical imperative for medical charity and the care of sick people, the importance of discernment between acceptable and unacceptable uses of spiritual methods in healing, and theological explanations of the origin and meaning of illness and bodily suffering.

The Protestant Reformation started as a religious movement with the primary intent of restoring the doctrinal alignment between medieval Catholic teachings on justification (or salvation) with those articulated in the New Testament, most prominently in the Pauline epistles. The Protestant program of doctrinal reform naturally and rapidly produced multiple implications for other important questions of Christian doctrine, practice, and ecclesial organization, as well as political, social, economic, and educational issues. With the excommunication of its intellectual founder, Martin Luther, from the Roman Catholic Church in 1521, Protestantism irreversibly took off as a third major form of the Christian religion. Starting in 1525, the Protestant movement itself began to split over internal disagreements among

Reformation leaders. Historians commonly distinguish between Magisterial reformers, like Luther, and Radical dissenters. Out of the Radical Reformation movement, various groups, including spiritualists and Anabaptists, subsequently emerged. Initially focused on a debate between Luther and his former ally, Andreas Bodenstein von Carlstadt, about the nature of the Eucharist, intra-Protestant disagreements were animated by deeper underlying religious differences pertaining to the relationship between the material and the spiritual. These differences had direct implications for religious debates about the proper place of the practice of medicine in the life of a Christian.

Luther saw the realm of physical matter as a conduit of God's work in the created world. Therefore, for Luther, certain material elements and objects, such as baptismal water, the bread and wine of the Eucharist, and the Bible, were to be valued and used as God's chosen vehicles of divine grace, as long as one maintained the proper perspective that it was God who ultimately exercised his supernatural power through the natural realm. This underlying theological perspective on materiality informed Luther's theology of medicine. Medicines were to be used gratefully as a gift from God, but not trusted in themselves. It was God who ultimately supplied healing through the use of medicine. At the same time, Luther opposed medieval Catholic devotional practices aimed at pursuing healing through the supernatural intercession of saints.

Luther's views on religion and medicine were expressed in his treatise *Whether One May Flee from a Deadly Plague* [7.1b]. Written during the 1527 outbreak of the Black Death, this pastoral letter defended the religious appropriateness of attempts to prevent and treat the disease against an attitude that the epidemic must not be resisted since it was a manifestation of God's punishment. This treatise also contained one of the most powerful examples of early Protestant engagement with the issue of medical service and an embrace of the Christian mandate to care self-sacrificially for sick people. In *The Babylonian Captivity of the Church* [7.1a], Luther expressed his position that scriptural promises of miraculous healings were primarily addressed to the early church and, therefore, generally no longer applied to his time.

Luther's theological perspectives on materiality and, by implication, on medicine, varied significantly from those of Carlstadt, Luther's former associate turned Radical reformer. Carlstadt's writings expressed a firm divide between the life-giving realm of the spirit and the realm of matter, deeming the latter, with the exception of the material records of scripture, as generally superfluous for higher spiritual purposes. Furthermore, Carlstadt, influenced by German medieval mysticism, insisted on the necessity of Christian abandonment (*Gelassenheit*) of the self, detachment from the world, and total yielding of desires to the will of God. This implied a detachment from pursuing and valuing certain material necessities, such as food and medicine, which is reflected in Carlstadt's 1523 treatise, *The Meaning of the Term Gelassen and Where in Holy Scripture It Is Found* [7.2]. Martin Luther's critique of such an attitude toward medicine is expressed, among other works, in his lectures on the biblical book of Isaiah [7.1d]. The theological appreciation of medicine by Magisterial Protestant reformers extended to giving high regard to the physician's profession as well as providing religious explanations for the possibilities of human medical knowledge and skill. In his *Sermon on Keeping Children at School* [7.1c], Luther spoke of society's great need for educated physicians and the divine establishment of the medical occupation.

In one of the greatest works of Protestant theological synthesis, *Institutes of the Christian Religion* [7.3b], John Calvin explained medical knowledge as God's gift to humanity, divinely transmitted to people even after they lost knowledge of the true God following Adam and Eve's radical disobedience (the Fall). One of the intellectual hallmarks of Calvin's theology was an emphasis on God's absolute sovereignty. Calvin rejected the notion of the divine "passive will," or God simply allowing certain events to happen. For Calvin, God's "active will" determined and regulated all human affairs, including human illnesses, incapacitations, and other instances of physical suffering. For example, in his *Commentary on a Harmony of the Evangelists, Matthew, Mark, and Luke* [7.3c], Calvin laid out his understanding of diseases as "heralds" of God's judgment. Such a position raises the question of why one should seek medical help if the outcome of one's illness is already immutably predetermined by God. The *Institutes* [7.3a] included Calvin's attempt to answer this question by presenting reasonable self-care as a Christian duty in submission to God's will. Furthermore, in *Commentary* [7.3d], Calvin offered a theological interpretation of the spiritual significance of Christ's physical healings.

As sixteenth-century theologians grappled with questions of medicine, physicians of that era drew on religion to explicate the meaning of their work. Protestants were not alone in their interest in questions of human and divine actions pertaining to medicine. The sixteenth-century French military doctor Ambroise Paré, a Catholic, is regarded by many as the father of modern surgery. In his *Journeys in Diverse Places* [7.4], Paré repeatedly described his work as merely the means through which God provided the cure—a reflection strikingly resembling Luther's understanding of medicine as a vehicle of God's work of healing. The famous medical iconoclast Paracelsus developed a curious fusion of medicine, alchemy, cosmology, magic, and unorthodox interpretations of Christianity. Paracelsus emphasized the centrality of chemistry for medical knowledge. He also adopted the ancient idea that the microcosm of a human body and soul reflected the composition of the cosmological macrocosm. Paracelsus's ideas about the divine ordination of the chemical composition of the universe are outlined in his *Philosophy Concerning the Generations of the Elements* [7.5].

Imagined modes of relating medicine and religion in the early modern era found expression in works of literature. For example, Girolamo Fracastoro, an accomplished physician, a former professor at the University of Padua, and the author of an insightful theory of the nature of contagion, wrote "Syphilis or the French Disease" [7.6]. This poem in Latin drew on classical mythology to create an origin myth for this new disease, which swept through Europe in the late fifteenth century. Fracastoro in many ways represented the intellectually multivalent Renaissance humanistic scholarship, as he combined in his poem imitations of classical myths with medical descriptions of the symptoms and treatments of syphilis.

Early modern controversies between Protestants and Catholics over what were spiritually acceptable methods of pursuing healing similarly found reflection in literary fiction. *The Anatomy of Melancholy* [7.7], written by Robert Burton, a seventeenth-century scholar at the University of Oxford and a clergyman of the Church of England, is an example. Its second "partition" discussed, from a Protestant perspective, questions about the religious legitimacy of various ways of treating melancholy (an umbrella term for mental disorders), the use of saintly intercession for healing, and the role of a physician. Although formally composed as a treatise on melancholy, its forms, and its possible cures, *The Anatomy of Melancholy* became famous for its extraordinary erudition in evoking numerous past and present medical and religious authorities, as well as for its satirical approach, which was ultimately skeptical about the very possibility of mental wellness.

Protestants were not the first to question certain medieval Catholic beliefs and practices pertaining to the search for healing. Long before the

Protestant Reformation, starting from the period of the mending of the Great Western Schism in the early 1400s, reform-minded individuals advocated (with varying degrees of success) addressing moral corruption and organizational abuses within the late medieval church, improving clerical education, and renewing lay devotional practices and Christian piety in society. Such sensibilities were realized in early modernity through a movement that took many forms and that is referred to by historians as the Catholic Reformation. Sixteenth-century Catholic reformers sought to distance themselves from their Protestant counterparts and their doctrinal agenda. Yet in their advocacy for the renewal of spiritual practices, including those pertaining to late medieval attitudes toward physical suffering and healing, these reformers often displayed concerns similar to those expressed by Protestants.

One of the intellectual leaders of the late fifteenth- and early sixteenth-century Catholic reform movement was the Dutch humanist Desiderius Erasmus. His famous work *Enchiridion* (or *The Handbook of the Militant Christian*) [7.8] criticized certain excesses of the medieval veneration of saints and the pursuits of their intercession for healing. However, the ultimate purposes of Erasmus's critique were different from those of Protestants, who tended to see the entire practice of seeking saintly assistance for healing as fundamentally idolatrous and therefore to think that they needed to be altogether abandoned. Erasmus instead advocated reforming certain aspects of and attitudes underlying such spiritual pursuits of bodily health. He challenged his readers to develop a deeper understanding of the reasons why they might employ spiritual means to seek bodily recovery, of the ultimate purpose and use of health in the Christian life, and of the centrality of Christ to the human pursuit of physical well-being.

Reform-minded concerns about certain medieval ascetic practices are found in the writings of Teresa of Ávila, a renowned sixteenth-century spiritual teacher in Spain. A new emphasis on the role of one's physical and mental ill-being in potentially negatively affecting one's spiritual experiences, along with a call for continuous sober discernment to avoid spiritual deception, characterized Teresa's discussions of spirituality and health in her mystical treatise *The Interior Castle* [7.9a]. Teresa is recognized for assigning equal importance to contemplation and action in monastic life. In the medieval West, action—including works of charity—had been viewed as essential yet inferior to contemplation, the devotional aspect of the monastic enterprise. In *The Interior Castle* [7.9b], the transformation of the hierarchy

of monastic duties was manifested in her emphasis on the spiritual significance of caring for sick people in monasteries.

Ignatius of Loyola was another profoundly significant early modern
Catholic reformer in Spain. Living through the beginning and rapid spread
of Protestantism, Ignatius accomplished much by developing distinctly
Catholic forms of spirituality and by promoting educational reform in the
troubled church through his influential devotional writings and the work of
the Society of Jesus (Jesuits), which he founded. Ignatius's *Autobiography*
[7.10a] described his own experience of serious injury as instrumental in his
conversion from a military career to the path of a religious life. His famed
devotional work *Spiritual Exercises* [7.10b] directed readers to employ bodily
practices to produce spiritual effects. At the beginning, the treatise laid out
the goal of achieving internal indifference toward one's condition, including the presence or absence of good health, in resignation to God's will. In
this way, the *Exercises* was an expression of the early modern propagation
of an ancient Christian spiritual tradition, conceivably influenced by ancient Stoic philosophy, that encouraged emotional detachment in matters of
one's physical well-being. Chapter 2 of the *Constitutions of the Society of
Jesus* [7.10c] addressed the question of preservation of health for the society's
members.

In Europe the long-standing tradition of clerical medicine and a perceived
Christian moral obligation to care for poor and sick people continued in new
forms into the age of Enlightenment, a period of increased public literacy
and popular distribution of knowledge. For example, the eighteenth-century
Church of England minister John Wesley, the founder of the Protestant
spiritual renewal movement that became known as Methodism, studied
medicine and established dispensaries for sick poor people. Wesley wrote
*Primitive Physick* [7.11], a collection of "safe and cheap and easy" natural
remedies for those who could not afford physicians' services. In Wesley's
native England, this self-help manual became one of the century's most
popular titles. The book opened with a religious explanation of the genesis
of disease, invoking the long-standing Christian tradition of tracing the
origin of illness to the Fall, before it outlined multiple natural remedies, while
still reminding readers of the centrality of religious devotion and prayer
to healing.

I close this chapter with examples of early modern non-Christian sources
that explored the relationship between religion and medicine, with particular attention to the moral duties of a doctor. The sixteenth-century "Maxim"

of Kung Hsin [7.12], which continued to influence Chinese medical ethics as late as the twentieth century, provided an ethical code for physicians in the Confucian tradition. A critique of the increasingly popular "professional" medicine from the standpoint of traditional Confucian principles is illustrated by the seventeenth-century *Chang's General Medicine* [7.13] by the Chinese physician Chang-Lu. One of the most renowned Jewish texts on the intersection of medicine and religion was the "Daily Prayer of a Physician" [7.14]. Traditionally attributed to Moses Maimonides, the prayer was first published about 1793 and was likely composed by the German physician Marcus Herz.

## TEXTS

### 7.1.
### Martin Luther

*Martin Luther (1483–1546), the German founder of the Protestant movement, was one of the most influential leaders in the history of Christianity. After years of living as a devout monk dedicated to the life of his order, scholarly studies, and the intense pursuit of pious living, Luther discovered in the Pauline epistles the teaching on justification by faith. In light of this discovery, Luther became convinced that the contemporary Catholic understanding of spiritual salvation, which required acts of virtue in addition to sincere faith in Jesus Christ, was erroneous and needed to be realigned with what he saw in scripture. Luther's exploration of the Bible led him to theologically scrutinize and challenge other established doctrines, ecclesial structures, and devotional practices.*

#### a. Sacrament of healing?
Martin Luther, *The Babylonian Captivity of the Church*[1]

*In his 1520 treatise, Luther critiqued the sacramental system of the Roman Catholic Church. He attacked the sacrament of extreme unction as founded on a misinterpretation of the teachings in the New Testament Epistle of James regarding miraculous healings.*

To the rite of anointing the sick our theologians have made two additions which are worthy of them; first, they call it a sacrament, and secondly, they make it the last sacrament. So that it is now the sacrament of extreme unction, which may be administered only to such as are at the point of death. Being such subtle dialecticians, perchance they have done this in order to relate it to the first unction of baptism and the two succeeding unctions of confirmation and ordination. But here they are able to cast in my teeth, that in the case of this sacrament there are, on the authority of James the Apostle, both promise and sign, which, as I have all along maintained, constitute a sacrament. For does not James say: (James 5:14f.) "Is any man sick among you? Let him bring in the priests of the church, and let them pray over him, anointing him with oil in the name of the Lord. And the prayer of faith shall raise him up: and if he be in sins, they shall be forgiven him." There, say they, you have the promise of the forgiveness of sins, and the sign of the oil. . . .

Furthermore, if this unction is a sacrament it must necessarily be, as they say, an effective sign of that which it signifies and promises. Now it promises health and recovery to the sick, as the words plainly say: "The prayer of faith shall save the sick man, and the Lord shall raise him up." But who does not see that this promise is seldom if ever fulfilled? Scarce one in a thousand is restored to health, and when one is restored nobody believes that it came about through the sacrament, but through the working of nature or the medicine; for to the sacrament they ascribe the opposite power. What shall we say then? Either the Apostle lies in making this promise or else this unction is no sacrament. For the sacramental promise is certain; but this promise deceives in the majority of cases. Indeed—and here again we recognize the shrewdness and foresight of these theologians—for this very reason they would have it to be extreme unction, that the promise should not stand; in other words, that the sacrament should be no sacrament. For if it is extreme unction, it does not heal, but gives way to the disease; but if it heals, it cannot be extreme unction. Thus, by the interpretation of these magisters, James is shown to have contradicted himself, and to have instituted a sacrament in order not to institute one; for they must have an extreme unction just to make untrue what the Apostle intends, namely, the healing of the sick. If that is not madness, pray what is?

Therefore, I take it, this unction is the same as that which the Apostles practiced, in Mark 6:13, "They anointed with oil many that were sick, and healed them." It was a ceremony of the early Church, by which they wrought miracles on the sick, and which has long since ceased; even as Christ, in the last chapter of Mark, gave them that believe the power to take up serpents, to lay hands on the sick, etc. (Mark 16:17). It is a wonder that they have not made sacraments also of these things; for they have the same power and promise as the words of James. Therefore, this extreme—that is, this fictitious—unction is not a sacrament, but a counsel of James, which whoever will may use, and it is derived from Mark 6, as I have shown. I do not believe it was a counsel given to all sick persons (Romans 5:3), for the Church's infirmity is her glory and death is gain (Philippians 1:21); but it was given only to such as might bear their sickness impatiently and with little faith. These the Lord allowed to remain in the Church, in order that miracles and the power of faith might be manifest in them.

### b. Caring for the sick during an epidemic
Martin Luther, *Whether One May Flee from a Deadly Plague*[2]

*This 1527 pastoral letter discussed a proper Christian response to the epidemic of plague.*

This I well know, that if it were Christ or his mother who were laid low by illness, everybody would be so solicitous and would gladly become a servant or helper. Everyone would want to be bold and fearless; nobody would flee but everyone would come running. And yet they don't hear what Christ himself says, "As you did to one of the least, you did it to me" [Matt. 25:40]. When he speaks of the greatest commandment he says, "The other commandment is like unto it, you shall love your neighbor as yourself" [Matt. 22:39]. There you hear that the command to love your neighbor is equal to the greatest commandment to love God, and that what you do or fail to do for your neighbor means doing the same to God. If you wish to serve Christ and to wait on him, very well, you have your sick neighbor close at hand. Go to him and serve him, and you will surely find Christ in him, not outwardly but in his word. If you do not wish or care to serve your neighbor you can be sure that if Christ lay there instead you would not do so either and would let him lie there. Those are nothing but illusions on your part which puff you up with vain pride, namely, that you would really serve Christ if he were there in person. Those are nothing but lies; whoever wants to serve Christ in person would surely serve his neighbor as well. This is said as an admonition and encouragement against fear and a disgraceful flight to which the devil would tempt us so that we would disregard God's command in our dealings with our neighbor and so we would fall into sin on the left hand.

Others sin on the right hand. They are much too rash and reckless, tempting God and disregarding everything which might counteract death and the plague. They disdain the use of medicines; they do not avoid places and persons infected by the plague, but lightheartedly make sport of it and wish to prove how independent they are. They say that it is God's punishment; if he wants to protect them he can do so without medicines or our carefulness. This is not trusting God but tempting him. God has created medicines and provided us with intelligence to guard and take good care of the body so that we can live in good health.

If one makes no use of intelligence or medicine when he could do so without detriment to his neighbor, such a person injures his body and must beware lest he become a suicide in God's eyes. By the same reasoning a person might forego eating and drinking, clothing and shelter, and boldly proclaim his faith that if God wanted to preserve him from starvation and cold, he could do so without food and clothing. Actually that would be suicide. It is even more shameful for a person to pay no heed to his own body and to fail to protect it against the plague the best he is able, and then to infect and poison others who might have remained alive if he had taken care of his body as he should have. He is thus responsible before God for his neighbor's death and is a murderer many times over. Indeed, such people behave as though a house were burning in the city and nobody were trying to put the fire out. Instead they give leeway to the flames so that the whole city is consumed, saying that if God so willed, he could save the city without water to quench the fire.

No, my dear friends, that is no good. Use medicine; take potions which can help you; fumigate house, yard, and street; shun persons and places wherever your neighbor does not need your presence or has recovered, and act like a man who wants to help put out the burning city. What else is the epidemic but a fire which instead of consuming wood and straw devours life and body? You ought to think this way: "Very well, by God's decree the enemy has sent us poison and deadly offal. Therefore I shall ask God mercifully to protect us. Then I shall fumigate, help purify the air, administer medicine, and take it. I shall avoid places and persons where my presence is not needed in order not to become contaminated and thus perchance infect and pollute others, and so cause their death as a result of my negligence. If God should wish to take me, he will surely find me and I have done what he has expected of me and so I am not responsible for either my own death or the death of others. If my neighbor needs me, however, I shall not avoid place or person but will go freely, as stated above." See, this is such a God-fearing faith because it is neither brash nor foolhardy and does not tempt God.

## c. Praise for physicians
Martin Luther, *Sermon on Keeping Children at School*[3]

*Luther's high regard for the medical vocation was expressed in this 1530 sermon.*

At this point I should also mention how many educated men are needed in the fields of medicine and the other liberal arts. Of these two needs one could write a huge book and preach for half a year. Where are the preachers, jurists, and physicians to come from, if grammar and other rhetorical arts are not taught? For such teaching is the spring from which they all must flow. . . .

We can see with our own eyes that the physicians are lords; experience teaches clearly that we cannot do without them. It is not the practice of medicine alone, however, but Scripture too that shows it to be a useful, comforting, and salutary estate, as well as a service acceptable to God, made and founded by him. In Ecclesiasticus 38[:1–8] almost an entire chapter is devoted to praise of the physicians, "Honor the physician, for one cannot do without him, and the Lord created him; for all healing comes from God."

## d. Use of but not reliance on medicine
Martin Luther, *Lectures on Isaiah*[4]

*As a professor at the University of Wittenberg, Luther lectured extensively on the Bible. This excerpt is from his lecture on Isaiah 38:1–21. The prophet Isaiah prescribed a poultice of figs to be applied to King Hezekiah's boil, despite having previously received God's promise that the king would recover. For Luther, the passage, while affirming the usefulness of a medical procedure, illustrated that it was not the medicine but God's promise (or Word) that produced recovery.*

Isaiah 38:21: Here Isaiah was made a physician. Here the physicians have their patron saint. For you heard in the song above that all things are kept and cared for by the Word. Then the ungodly cry: "If the Word does everything and provides nourishment for everything, we do not want to eat or take medicine." For them he takes up this example. As for you, make use of means. Do not rely on them but use them, since God has created them. If they do not help, commit the matter to God. Do not say: "Doctor, if this will not help this time, I refuse to take it anymore." Yes, you want to have your own way! So we all go beyond the proper use of means by clinging to them, as our papists altogether cling to works. Others despise works altogether, so does this song ascribe the power to the Word and not to the medicine. Yet it does not forbid that we use them, but the prophet's example supports their use, since he poultices the wound with a cake of figs. Therefore we must make use of means. We must work and produce and commit ourselves to God.

## 7.2
### Against trust in medicine
Andreas Carlstadt, *The Meaning of the Term Gelassen and Where in Holy Scripture It Is Found*[5]

*Andreas Bodenstein von Carlstadt (1486–1541) was a German theologian and Radical reformer with strong mystical inclinations. His works had an important impact on the early Anabaptist movement. Carlstadt and Luther's theological camaraderie was shattered after the former undertook a series of reforms in Wittenberg during Luther's incognito stay in the castle of Wartburg from 1520 to 1521. In 1523, Carlstadt left his University of Wittenberg professorship for a parish church in Orlamünde. During this time Carlstadt published, under the pseudonym the New Layman, the treatise excerpted here, which was significantly influenced by medieval German mystical theologies. Carlstadt's attitude toward food and medicine was part of his theological insistence on the necessity of Christians' surrender or "yieldedness" of all aspects of their lives to the will and provision of God.*

If we had the right faith in God and trusted God with all our hearts and knew God to be our Father who cares more diligently about us than we ourselves and never feeds us less than the unreasoning animals, we would be without care and yielding with regard to food. . . .

The Yieldedness of Intellect: Human beings have intellect which enables them to be wise and to plan ahead. It allows them to build cities and houses, to make weapons and all kinds of protection. This leads people to become rather unyielded when they ought to leave shelter and protection to God and not to seek more. I could demonstrate this by reference to several prophets, but I won't for the sake of brevity, and merely refer to what God says, "You put your trust in your own defenses which you made for yourselves" (Jeremiah 48:7; Isaiah 2:11, 17; 9:5; 16:8; 31:3). Therefore God will forsake you and surrender you to your enemies. Thus many princes and warriors were destroyed who might otherwise have survived and recovered before God.

I should also mention at this point that David took no comfort in a bow or sword, but killed Goliath with a slingshot. That is a simple matter and not worth writing about. But the sick should take notice who put a deceptive trust in doctors and herbal medicine (2 Chronicles 16:12).

Hence, all external things are to be clearly avoided and yielded, so that they might not deceive us.

## 7.3
## John Calvin

*John Calvin (1509–1564), a second-generation Magisterial Protestant reformer from France, was a founder of what later became known as the Reformed tradition in Protestant Christianity. He was an ecclesiastical organizer in the Swiss town of Geneva and a deeply influential and prolific theological thinker, writer, and preacher.*

### a. Divine providence and human responsibility
### in caring for one's health
John Calvin, *Institutes of the Christian Religion*[6]

*At the age of twenty-seven, Calvin published the first edition of his most important work,* Institutes of the Christian Religion. *Calvin continued to revise and extend this work, which became one of the most significant Protestant theological syntheses. He intended to systematically articulate and defend the main tenets of Protestant faith. The following two passages from the final 1559 edition of the* Institutes *address God's providence vis-à-vis human responsibility in matters of health care, and medical knowledge as a divine gift to undeserving humanity, even to those who do not recognize God as the true source of this knowledge.*

Profane men, with their absurdities foolishly raise an uproar, so that they almost, as the saying is, mingle heaven and earth. If the Lord has indicated the point of our death, they say, we cannot escape it. Therefore it is vain for anyone to busy himself in taking precautions. One man does not dare take a road that he hears is dangerous, lest he be murdered by thieves; another summons physicians, and wears himself out with medicines to keep himself alive; another abstains from coarser foods, lest he impair his weak health; another is afraid of living in tumble-down houses. Now [they conclude] either all these remedies which attempt to correct God's will are vain; or else there is no fixed decree of God that determines life and death, health and disease, peace and war, and other things that men, as they desire or hate them, so earnestly try by their own toil either to obtain or to avoid. . . .

But with respect to future events, Solomon easily brings human deliberations into agreement with God's providence. For just as he laughs at the dullness of those who boldly undertake something or other without the Lord, as though they were not ruled by his hand, so elsewhere he says: "Man's heart plans his way, but the Lord will direct his steps" [Prov. 16:9]. This means that we are not at all hindered by God's eternal decrees either from looking ahead for ourselves or from putting all our affairs in order, but always in submission to his will. The reason is obvious. For he who has set the limits to our life has at the same time entrusted to us its care; he has provided means and helps to preserve it; he has also made us able to foresee dangers; that they may not overwhelm us unaware, he has offered precautions and remedies. Now it is very clear what our duty is: thus, if the Lord has committed to us the protection of our life, our duty is to protect it; if he offers helps, to use them; if he forewarns us of dangers, not to plunge headlong; if he makes remedies available, not to neglect them.

### b. Medicine as a divine gift
John Calvin, *Institutes of the Christian Religion*[7]

Whenever we come upon these matters in secular writers, let that admirable light of truth shining in them teach us that the mind of man, though fallen and perverted from its wholeness, is nevertheless clothed and ornamented with God's excellent gifts. If we regard the Spirit of God as the sole fountain of truth, we shall neither reject the truth itself, nor despise it wherever it shall appear, unless we wish to dishonor the Spirit of God. For by holding the gifts of the Spirit in slight esteem, we condemn and reproach the Spirit himself. What then? Shall we deny that the truth shone upon the ancient jurists who established civic order and discipline with such great equity? Shall we say that the philosophers were blind in their fine observation and artful description of nature? Shall we say that those men were devoid of understanding who conceived the art of disputation and taught us to speak reasonably? Shall we say that they are insane who developed medicine, devoting their labor to our benefit?

. . .

No, we cannot read the writings of the ancients on these subjects without great admiration. We marvel at them because we are compelled to recognize how preeminent they are. But shall we count anything praiseworthy or noble without recognizing at the same time that it comes from God? Let us be ashamed of such ingratitude, into which not even the pagan poets fell, for they confessed that the gods had invented philosophy, laws, and all useful arts. Those men whom Scripture [1 Cor. 2:14] calls "natural men" were, indeed, sharp and penetrating in their investigation of inferior things. Let us, accordingly, learn by their example how many gifts the Lord left to human nature even after it was despoiled of its true good.

### c. *Diseases as heralds of God's judgment*
John Calvin, *Commentary on a Harmony of the Evangelists,*
*Matthew, Mark, and Luke*[8]

*In the following excerpts from this commentary published in 1555, Calvin offered his interpretation of Luke 4:39 ("He rebuked the fever") and of Matthew 8:17 ("That it might be fulfilled which was spoken by Isaiah the prophet, when he saith, 'He hath taken our sicknesses and hath carried our diseases'") as referring to Jesus's ministry.*

Luke 4:39. *He {Jesus} rebuked the fever.* To a person not well acquainted with Scripture this mode of expression may appear harsh; but there were good reasons for employing it. Fevers and other diseases, famine, pestilence, and calamities of every description, are God's heralds, by whom he executes his judgments. Now, as he is said to send such messengers by his command and pleasure, so he also restrains and recalls them whenever he pleases.

### d. *Spiritual significance of Jesus's healings*
John Calvin, *Commentary on a Harmony of the Evangelists,*
*Matthew, Mark, and Luke*[9]

Matthew 8:17: *That it might be fulfilled which was spoken by Isaiah the prophet.* . . . What is undoubtedly spoken about the impurities of the soul, Matthew applies to bodily diseases. The solution is not difficult, if the reader will only observe, that the Evangelist states not merely the benefit conferred by Christ on those sick persons, but the purpose for which he healed their diseases. They experienced in their bodies the grace of Christ, but we must look at the design: for it would be idle to confine our view to a transitory advantage, as if the Son of God were a physician of bodies. What then? He gave sight to the blind, in order to show that he is "the light of the world" (John 8:12). He restored life to the dead, to prove that he is "the resurrection and the life" (John 11:25). Similar observations might be made as to those who were lame, or had palsy. Following out this analogy, let us connect those benefits, which Christ bestowed on men in the flesh, with the design which is stated to us by Matthew, that he was sent by the Father, to relieve us from all evils and miseries.

## 7.4
## Divine and human agency in medicine
Ambroise Paré, *Journeys in Diverse Places*[10]

*Ambroise Paré (1510–1590), a surgeon to four French kings, is often considered the founder of modern surgery and military medicine. Among Paré's most influential accomplishments were introducing new practices for treating gunshot wounds, reviving an old method of tying rather than cauterizing arteries during surgery, and using ligatures for limb amputations, which allowed for the amputation of thighs. With the increase in gunshot injuries in warfare, such treatments became increasingly essential to save lives. "I dressed him, and God healed him" is a recurrent theme in Paré's 1585* Journeys, *which described his field observations and experiences as a traveling surgeon.*

All the seigneurs within the town asked me to give special care, above all the rest, to M. de Pienne, who had been wounded, while on the breach, by a stone shot from a cannon, on the temple, with fracture and depression of the bone. They told me that so soon as he received the blow, he fell to the ground as dead, and cast forth blood by the mouth, nose, and ears, with great vomiting, and was fourteen days without being able to speak or reason; also he had tremors of a spasmodic nature, and all his face was swelled and livid. He was trepanned at the side of the temporal muscle, over the frontal bone. I dressed him, with other surgeons, and God healed him; and today he is still living, thank God.

## 7.5
## Chemical composition of cosmology
Paracelsus, *Philosophy Concerning the Generations of the Elements*[11]

*Paracelsus (1493–1541), born Philippus Aureolus Theophrastus Bombastus von Hohenheim, was a German physician and alchemist. A Catholic with Radical Reformation sympathies, he was praised by some as the "Luther of science" and denounced by others as a magician and heretic. Paracelsus was famous for his disdain for traditional medical authorities and his emphasis on the study of nature. He produced an original theory of disease and promoted the role of chemistry in medicine. The following excerpt describes the divine creation of the chemical composition of the universe. "Iliaster" was Paracelsus's term for a primeval substance encompassing both matter and spirit.*

Now, in order to advance towards the established principle with regard to the elements, understand this. The Iliaster was originally distributed into four parts—the air, which is a heaven embracing all things; fire, which is a firmament producing day and night, cold and heat; earth, which affords fruits of all kinds and a solid foundation for our feet; and water from whence are given forth all minerals and half the means of nutriment for living things. These nutriments are twofold, one found in air and fire, the other in earth and water. The two former nourish us as if spiritually and invisibly; the two latter materially and corporeally. . . .

It should be known, then, at the outset, and before the philosophy itself is unfolded, that God has made the center of His heaven, and even Himself, perishable. For as corporeally He is called the Son, so the world is His house. But although it be thus made and created, still we must believe that it will not perish as it was produced. Of man the heart will endure: of the world the flower will be permanent.

As to the manner in which God created the world, take the following account. He originally reduced it to one body, while the elements were developing. This body He made up of three ingredients, Mercury, Sulphur, and Salt, so that these three should constitute one body. Of these three are composed all the things which are, or are produced, in the four elements. . . .

First of all He produced and separated the air. This being formed, from the remainder issued forth the other three elements, fire, water, earth. From these He afterwards took away the fire, while the other two remained, and so on in due succession.

## 7.6
## Medicine and religion in literary arts I
Girolamo Fracastoro, "Syphilis or the French Disease"[12]

*Girolamo Fracastoro (c. 1478–1553) was an Italian humanist, physician, philosopher, and poet. The following excerpt is from his 1530 poem "Syphilis or the French Disease," which coined the name of the illness. This mythical medical epic in three books was the story of a fictional shepherd named Syphilus, the first victim of the disease. Syphilus was struck by the sun god for abandoning his worship in favor of giving divine honors to a mortal king, Alcithous.*

Syphilus, a shepherd by this very river, so the story goes, used to pasture a thousand oxen and a thousand snow-white sheep over these pastures for king Alcithous: the time was just at the summer solstice; Sirius was scorching the thirsty fields, was scorching the groves; and the woods offered no shade to shepherds, the wind offered no relief. He pitied his flock, and provoked by the fierce heat lifted up his eyes and face to the Sun in its eminence. "Why, Sun, do we call you Father and God of all things and why do we, the ignorant masses, lay out sacred altars and worship you with sacrifice of ox and casket rich in incense, if you have no concern for us and the king's flocks do not touch your heart? Or rather am I to think that you Gods are scorched with envy? By me a thousand cattle, white as snow, are pastured, by me a thousand sheep; you have in heaven, if reports are true, merely one Bull, one Ram—and one dried-up Bitch to guard this enormous herd. What a fool I am, that I don't rather perform divine rites for the king, who has so many estates, so many subjects, whom the broad seas supply and whose power is greater than the Gods and the Sun. The king will grant favouring breezes, he will bring the sweet coolness of green groves to our herds and lighten the burden of the heat." So he spoke; no delay; he set up sacred altars on the mountains to king Alcithous and performed divine rites. This the hosts of country folk followed, this the rest of the shepherd crowd; they burnt offerings of incense at their hearths and they made offerings of bull's blood, and roasted the steaming entrails. When the king heard of this while he happened to be seated on his throne amid a packed crowd of his subject peoples, delighted by the honour due to Gods being shown to him, he decreed that no other godly power should be worshipped on earth, or he would exact punishment; on the world itself nothing was greater than him; the Gods lived in the sky, what lay below was not theirs. He had seen these events, who sees all things, who reviews all things in detail, the Sun the Father, and he felt indignation in his mind, he hurled his hostile rays and shone with a bitter light. By that glance mother Earth and the sea's flat expanse were attacked, by that venom the air was infected and began to glow hot. Straightway an unknown pollution was born to flood the blasphemous earth. The first man to display disfiguring sores over his body was Syphilus, who by the shedding of blood instituted divine rites in the king's honour and altars in the mountains sacred to him; he was the first to experience sleepless nights and tortured limbs, and from this very first victim the disease derived its name and from him the farmers called the sickness Syphilis.

### 7.7
### Medicine and religion in literary arts II
Robert Burton, *The Anatomy of Melancholy*[13]

*Robert Burton (1577–1640) was the librarian of Christ Church College at Oxford and a clergyman of the Church of England. In 1621, he published* The Anatomy of Melancholy, *a satirical Protestant medical work, under the pseudonym Democritus Junior. (The ancient Greek Democritus was known as "the laughing philosopher.") The book was a success, went through five subsequent editions in Burton's lifetime, and earned high praise from some of England's most renowned authors. The following passage is from the second of three "partitions" of this volume, which distinguished between "unlawful"—and therefore religiously unacceptable—and "lawful" cures for melancholy.*

That we must pray to God, no man doubts; but whether we should pray to saints in such cases, or whether they can do us any good, it may be lawfully controverted. Whether their images, shrines, relics, consecrated things, holy water, medals, benedictions, those divine amulets, holy exorcisms, and the sign of the cross, be available in this disease? The papists on the one side stiffly maintain how many melancholy, mad, demoniacal persons are daily cured at St. Anthony's Church in Padua, at St. Vitus' in Germany, by our Lady of Loretto in Italy, our Lady of Sichem in the Low Countries. . . . They have a proper saint almost for every peculiar infirmity: for poison, gouts, agues, Petronella: St. Romanus for such as are possessed; Valentine for the falling sickness; St. Vitus for madmen. . . .

But we on the other side seek to God alone. We say with David (Psal. xlvi.1) "God is our hope and strength, and help in trouble, ready to be found." For their catalogue of examples, we make no other answer, but that they are false fictions, or diabolical illusions, counterfeit miracles. We cannot deny but that it is an ordinary thing on St. Anthony's day in Padua, to bring diverse madmen and demoniacal persons to be cured: yet we make a doubt whether such parties be so affected indeed, but prepared by their priests, by certain ointments and drams, to cozen the commonalty. . . .

But we need not run so far for examples in this kind, we have a just volume published at home to this purpose, "A declaration of egregious popish impostures, to withdraw the hearts of religious men under the pretense of casting out of devils, practiced by Father Edmunds, alias Weston, a Jesuit, and divers Romish priests, his wicked associates," with the several parties' names, confessions, examinations, etc. which were pretended to be possessed. But these are ordinary tricks only to get opinion and money, mere impostures. Aesculapius of old, that counterfeit God, did as many famous cures; his temple (as Strabo relates) was daily full of patients, and as many several tables, inscriptions, pendants, donories, etc. to be seen in his church, as at this day at our Lady of Loretto's in Italy. It was a custom long since, to do the like, in former times they were seduced and deluded as they are now. 'Tis the same devil still, called heretofore Apollo, Mars, Neptune, Venus, Aesculapius, etc. (as Lactantius *lib. 2. de orig. erroris, c. 17.* observes), the same Jupiter and those bad angels are now worshipped and adored by the name of St. Sebastian, Barbara, Christopher and George are come in their places. . . .

Why should we rather seek to them, than to Christ himself, since that he so kindly invites us unto him, "Come unto me all ye that are heavy laden, and I will ease you" (Mat. xi), and we know that there is one God, "one Mediator between God and man, Jesus Christ" (1 Tim. ii.5), "who gave himself a ransom for all men."

## 7.8
### Medicine and Catholic moral reform
Desiderius Erasmus, *Enchiridion*[14]

*Desiderius Erasmus (c. 1467–1536), a Dutch Catholic humanist scholar, is remembered as the leading intellectual of the northern Renaissance, a moralist, satirist, translator, educational reformer, and prolific writer. Born to an unwed*

*mother, a start in life promising challenges in early modernity, Erasmus even-*
*tually gained widespread European recognition for his extraordinary learned-*
*ness and intellectual accomplishments. Erasmus's two central aspirations*
*were humanist educational reform through a revival of classical education and*
*moral reform of the church through addressing structural abuses and encour-*
*aging Christian piety. The following excerpt is from his 1503* Enchiridion (*or*
The Handbook of the Militant Christian), *written with the latter end in mind.*
*After being reprinted in 1518, the* Enchiridion *became an extremely popular book*
*of spiritual instruction and was translated into many languages.*

Suppose you decide to fast. Certainly this has all the appearance of a virtuous act. But what is the motive for your fasting; to what do you refer it? Is it
not perhaps that you might conserve food? Is it because others will then
think you more pious? Most likely you fast in order to preserve your health.
And why are you fearful of overeating? For the simple reason that this can
interfere with your pursuit of pleasure. Perhaps you are concerned about
your health so that you can continue your studies. And why, might I ask, are
you so concerned about studies? In order to obtain the easy living of a clergyman, living that is really for your own pleasure and not for Christ's. You
have really missed the target toward which every Christian ought to aim. If
you can eat sufficiently and take care of your health so that you can take
part in religious exercises, then you are hitting the mark. If your concern
for health and gracious living is only to enable you to be more vigorous in
lustful pursuits, you have fallen away from Christ and have made a god out
of yourself.

Now there are not a few who are given over to the veneration of the
saints, with elaborate ceremonies. Some, for example, have a great devotion
to St. Christopher. Provided his statue is in sight, they pray to him almost
every day. Why do they do this? It is because they wish to be preserved from
a sudden and unprovided-for death that day. There are others who have a
great devotion to St. Roch. Why? Because they believe that Roch can immu-
nize them against certain physical ailments. Others mumble certain prayers
to St. Barbara or St. George so they will not fall into the hands of the enemy.
Still others fast in honor of St. Apollo so that they will not be troubled with
toothaches. Others visit the image of holy Job to prevent boils. There are
certain merchants who assign a portion of their profits to the poor so that
they will not suffer a loss of merchandise in shipwreck. A candle is burned
in honor of St. Jerome so that lost goods might be recovered. In short, for

everything we fear or desire we set up a corresponding deity. This has gone to the extent that each nation has its own. Among the French St. Paul is esteemed, among us Germans St. Jerome has a special place. Certain areas hold St. James or St. John in lesser or greater esteem. This kind of piety, since it does not refer either our fears or our desires to Christ, is hardly a Christian practice. As a matter of fact, it is not a great deal different from the superstitions of the ancients. They pledged a tenth of their goods to Hercules that they might get rich, or a cock to Aesculapius to regain their health. A bull was sacrificed to Neptune to avoid mishap at sea. The names may have changed, but the purpose and intentions are the same. . . .

I am sure that these remarks will be disturbing to certain so-called saintly men who identify the worship of God with financial gain and who, with their sweet benedictions, deceive the minds of the innocent, serving their own bellies rather than Christ. They will protest that I am forbidding the veneration of the saints in whom God is also honored. I do not damn those who do such things with a simple and childish sort of superstition so much as I do those who, for their own advantage, magnify these practices completely out of proportion. They encourage these devotions, which of themselves are tolerable, for their own profit and thereby capitalize on the ignorance of the masses. What I utterly condemn is the fact that they esteem the indifferent in place of the highest, the nonessentials to the complete neglect of what is essential. What is of the smallest value spiritually they make the greatest. I will certainly praise them for seeking a healthy body from St. Roch, provided they consecrate their life to Christ. But I will praise them still more if they pray for nothing else than a love of virtue and of hatred for vice. As for dying or living, let them leave such matters in the hands of God, and let them say with Paul, "Whether we live, we live unto the Lord; and whether we die, we die unto the Lord." What would be ideal is that they desire to be dissolved from the body and be with Christ. It would be perfect if they, in disease and misfortune, make their real joy consist in this, that they have conformed their lives to Christ their head. Accordingly, to practice these devotions is not so much to be condemned as is the danger inherent in them, namely, that of relying entirely or too much on them. I suffer from infirmity and weakness, but with St. Paul I show forth a more excellent way. Examine yourself in light of these rules and you will not be content with these indifferent actions until all of them are referred to Christ; you will not stop midway but will continue so that all is aimed at serving and honoring God.

## 7.9
## Teresa of Ávila

*St. Teresa of Ávila (1515–1582) was a Spanish spiritual teacher, mystical theologian, and monastic reformer. Having joined a Carmelite convent at the age of twenty-one, Teresa initially led a semisecular life, which was not uncommon during that era for aristocratic offspring entering monastic institutions. Teresa gradually became convinced of the necessity of stricter forms of piety and started to have mystical experiences. She labored for the spiritual reform of Carmelite monastic life and personally established fifteen houses for women, guided two from a distance, and assisted in founding two communities for men. She is considered one of the most significant writers during Spain's Golden Age. Canonized forty years after her death, Teresa of Ávila became, in the twentieth century, the first woman formally recognized as a doctor of the Roman Catholic Church. Her 1577 work,* The Interior Castle, *was written as a mystical spiritual directive to the soul progressing toward a spiritual union with God.*

### a. Health and monastic spirituality
Teresa of Ávila, *The Interior Castle*[15]

*This passage discusses the intersection of the physical and the spiritual in the context of monastic spirituality. It reflected Teresa's pervasive concern with spiritual deception and false spiritual experiences, which she saw as possibly caused by physical or mental disorders in some cases. "Favor" and "consolation" referred to intense spiritual experiences of divine proximity and love, which were achieved through prayer and may even have brought one to the state of physical exhaustion known as "spiritual sleep."*

There is one danger I want to warn you about (although I may have mentioned it elsewhere) into which I have seen persons of prayer fall, especially women, for since we are weaker there is more occasion for what I'm about to say. It is that some have a weak constitution because of a great amount of penance, prayer, and keeping vigil, and even without these; in receiving some favor, their nature is overcome. Since they feel some consolation interiorly and a languishing and weakness exteriorly, they think they are experiencing a spiritual sleep (which is a prayer a little more intense than the prayer of quiet) and they let themselves become absorbed. The more they allow this, the more absorbed they become because their nature is further weakened, and they fancy that they are being carried away in rapture. I call it being carried away in foolishness because it amounts to nothing more than wasting time and wearing down one's health. These persons feel nothing through their senses nor do they feel anything concerning God. One person happened to remain eight hours in this state. By sleeping and eating and avoiding so much penance, this person got rid of the stupor, for there was someone who understood her. She had misled both her confessor and other persons, as well as herself—for she hadn't intended to deceive. I truly believe that the devil was trying to gain ground, and in this instance indeed he was beginning to gain no small amount. . . .

The prioress should make them {such nuns} give up so many hours for prayer so that they have only a very few and try to get them to sleep and eat well until their natural strength begins to return, if it has been lost through a lack of food and sleep. If a Sister's nature is so weak that this is not enough, may she believe me that God does not want her to practice anything but the active life, which also must be practiced in monasteries. They should let her get busy with different duties, and always take care that she not have a great deal of solitude, for she would lose her health completely.

### b. Contemplation and healing action
Teresa of Ávila, *The Interior Castle*[16]

*This excerpt emphasizes the spiritual importance of care for sick people. "Union" referred to the state of radical conformity of the Christian's will to God's will.*

When I see souls very earnest in trying to understand the prayer they have and very sullen when they are in it—for it seems they don't dare let their minds move or stir lest a bit of their spiritual delight and devotion be lost—it makes me realize how little they understand of the way by which union is attained; they think the whole matter lies in these things. No, Sisters, absolutely not; works are what the Lord wants. He desires that if you see a Sister who is sick to whom you can bring some relief, you have compassion on her and not worry about losing this devotion; and that if she is suffering pain, you also feel it; and that, if necessary, you fast so that she might eat—not so much for her sake as because you know it is your Lord's desire. This is true union with His will.

## 7.10
## Ignatius of Loyola

*St. Ignatius of Loyola (c. 1491–1556), the founder of the Society of Jesus (Jesuits), was a spiritual writer, teacher, and Catholic ecclesial organizer. Having initially prepared for a military career, Ignatius was seriously wounded at the siege of Pamplona, was thereafter converted, and embarked on a life of religious devotion.*

### a. Conversion through illness
Ignatius of Loyola, *Autobiography*[17]

*Ignatius described his conversion in his* Autobiography, *which he dictated between 1553 and 1555. Ignatius spoke about himself in the third person. During a time of physical recovery Ignatius first underwent spiritual experiences he later identified as desolation and consolation. Attentiveness to these internal motions became crucial for his most significant theological work,* Spiritual Exercises.

And his bones having knit together, one bone below the knee was left riding on another, which made the leg shorter. The bone protruded so much that it was an ugly business. He could not bear such a thing because he was set on a worldly career and thought that this would deform him; he asked the surgeons if it could be cut away. They said that it could indeed be cut away, but that the pain would be greater than all that he had suffered, because it was already healed and it would take a while to cut it. And yet he chose on his own to make himself a martyr, though his elder brother was shocked and said that he himself would not dare suffer such pain; but the wounded man bore it with his wonted endurance.

After the flesh and excess bone were cut away, remedial measures were taken that the leg might not be so short. Ointment was often applied, and it was stretched continually with instruments that tortured him for many days. But Our Lord kept giving him health, and he felt so well that he was quite fit except that he could not stand easily on his leg and had perforce to stay in bed.

As he was much given to reading worldly books of fiction, commonly labeled chivalry, when he felt better he asked to be given some of them to pass the time. But in that house none of those that he usually read could be found, so they gave him a life of Christ and a book of the lives of saints in Castilian. . . .

When he was thinking of those things of the world he took much delight in them, but afterwards, when he was tired and put them aside, he found himself dry and dissatisfied. But when he thought of going to Jerusalem barefoot, and of eating nothing but plain vegetables and of practicing all the other rigors that he saw in the saints, not only was he consoled when he had these thoughts, but even after putting them aside he remained satisfied and joyful.

### b. Internal indifference in matters of health
Ignatius of Loyola, *Spiritual Exercises*[18]

*Developed over a span of twenty-five years,* Spiritual Exercises *was printed in 1548 as a program of personal spiritual growth. This passage is from the opening part of this work, outlining the ultimate goal of a Christian life.*

Man was created for this end, that he might praise and reverence the Lord his God, and, serving Him, save his soul.

But the other things which are placed on the earth were created for man's sake, that they might assist him in pursuing the end of his creation: whence it follows, that they are to be used or abstained from in proportion as they profit or hinder him in pursuing that end.

Wherefore we ought to be indifferent towards all created things (in so far as it is left to the freedom of our will, and not prohibited), so that (to the best of our power) we seek not health more than sickness, nor prefer riches to poverty, honor to contempt, a long life to a short one.

But it is fitting, out of all, to choose and desire those things only which lead us to the end for the sake of which we were created.

### c. Active preservation of the body
Ignatius of Loyola, *Constitutions of the Society of Jesus*[19]

*This passage from the* Constitutions *set moderation as the standard in the preservation of personal health for Jesuits.*

Just as an excessive preoccupation over the needs of the body is blameworthy, so too a proper concern about the preservation of one's health and bodily strength for the divine service is praiseworthy, and all should exercise it.

## 7.11
## Healthy lifestyle
John Wesley, *Primitive Physick*[20]

*John Wesley (1703–1791) was a priest in the Church of England and the founder of Methodism, an evangelical Protestant movement that emphasized God's love for all people, high standards of personal piety, and social service. The following excerpt is from the preface of Wesley's 1747* Primitive Physick; or, An Easy and Natural Method of Curing Most Diseases. *The book was composed as a self-help manual, an increasingly popular genre in Enlightenment England. It contained natural remedies and health-care advice that were accessible and affordable for poor and undereducated people.*

When man came first out of the hands of the great Creator, clothed in body as well as in soul, with immortality and incorruption, there was no place for physic, or the art of healing. As he knew no sin, so he knew no pain, no sickness, weakness, or bodily disorder. The habitation wherein the angelic mind, the *Divinae particula aurae* [particle of the divine light] abode, though originally formed out of the dust of the earth, was liable to no decay. It had no seeds of corruption or dissolution within itself. And there was nothing without to injure it: Heaven and earth and all the hosts of them were mild, benign, and friendly to human nature. The entire creation was at peace with man, so long as man was at peace with his Creator. So that well might "the morning stars sing together, and all the sons of God shout for joy."

But since man rebelled against the Sovereign of heaven and earth, how entirely is the scene changed! The incorruptible frame hath put on corruption, the immortal has put on mortality. The seeds of weakness and pain, of sickness and death, are now lodged in our inmost substance; whence a thousand disorders continually spring, even without the aid of external violence. And how is the number of these increased by every thing round about us! The heavens, the earth, and all things contained therein, conspire to punish the rebels against their Creator. The sun and moon shed unwholesome influences from above; the earth exhales poisonous damps from beneath; the beasts of the field, the birds of the air, the fishes of the sea, are in a state of hostility: yea, the food we eat, daily saps the foundation of the life which cannot be sustained without it. So has the Lord of all secured the execution of his decrees,—"Dust thou art, and unto dust thou shalt return."

But can there nothing be found to lessen those inconveniences, which cannot be wholly removed? To soften the evils of life, and prevent in part the sickness and pain to which we are continually exposed? Without question there may. One grand preventative of pain and sickness of various kinds, seems intimated by the great Author of nature in the very sentence that entails death upon us: "In the sweat of thy face shalt thou eat bread, 'till thou return to the ground." The power of exercise, both to preserve and restore health, is greater than can well be conceived; especially in those who add temperance thereto; who if they do not confine themselves altogether to eat either "bread or the herb of the field" (which God does not require them to do), yet steadily observe both that kind and measure of food, which experience shews to be most friendly to health and strength. . . .

As to the manner of using the medicines here set down, I should advise. . . .

Observe all the time the greatest exactness in your regimen or manner of living. Abstain from all mixed, all high seasoned food. Use plain diet, easy of digestion; and this as sparingly as you can, consistent with ease and strength. Drink only water, if it agrees with your stomach; if not, good, clear small beer. Use as much exercise daily in the open air, as you can without weariness. Sup at six or seven on the lightest food; go to bed early, and rise betimes. To persevere with steadiness in this course, is often more than half the cure. Above all, add to the rest (for it is not labour lost), that old unfashionable medicine, prayer. And have faith in God who "killeth and maketh alive, who bringeth down to the grace, and bringeth up."

## 7.12
## Confucian views of a good physician I
### Kung Hsin, "Maxim"[21]

*Kung Hsin was a sixteenth-century Confucian physician at the Chinese imperial court who authored several medical treatises. His "Maxim" (c. 1556) provided concise guidelines for the ethical conduct of physicians, together with praise for the impact of a virtuous doctor. This text, influential in the history of Chinese medicine, was introduced in 1939 as part of the baccalaureate ceremony at Peiping Union Medical College.*

The good physician of the present day cherishes kindness and righteousness. He reads widely and is highly skilled in the arts of his profession. He has in his mind adequate methods of treatment, which he adapts to different conditions. He cares not for vainglory, but is intent upon relieving suffering among all classes. He revives the dying and restores them to health: his beneficence is equal to that of Providence. Such a good physician will be remembered through endless generations.

**7.13**
### Confucian views of a good physician II
Chang-Lu, *Chang's General Medicine*[22]

*Chang-Lu (1627–1707) was a Confucian physician, author, and publisher of several medical works. Although it is unknown whether he ever passed Confucian examinations, Chang-Lu was concerned with the departure of contemporary medicine from the traditional orthodox Confucian paradigm. In the first chapter of his 1695 treatise,* Chang's General Medicine, *he outlined ten prohibitions for physicians, summarized in the excerpt below. Particularly notable are the prohibitions of practicing magical (or religiously heterodox) healing and treating noble and common patients similarly, the latter being justified by the assertion that noble patients were more physically fragile.*

(The physician shall abstain from):
Acquiring evil habits
Over self-confidence
Strong prejudice
Imitation or lack of initiative
Making careless diagnosis
Practicing magic healing
Treating the nobility and commoners similarly
Neglecting poor patients
Extorting high compensation from critical cases
Criticizing or slandering other physicians.

## 7.14
## Judaism and medicine
### "Daily Prayer of a Physician"[23]

*The "Daily Prayer of a Physician" was first published around 1793 under the title "Daily Prayer of a Physician before He Visits His Patients—from the Hebrew Manuscript of a Famous Jewish Physician in Egypt of the Twelfth Century." Although traditionally attributed to Moses Maimonides, the prayer is now considered by many to have been written in the eighteenth century by the Jewish doctor Marcus Herz.*

Almighty God, Thou has created the human body with infinite wisdom. Ten thousand times ten thousand organs hast Thou combined in it that act unceasingly and harmoniously to preserve the whole in all its beauty the body which is the envelope of the immortal soul. They are ever acting in perfect order, agreement and accord. Yet, when the frailty of matter or the unbridling of passions deranges this order or interrupts this accord, then forces clash and the body crumbles into the primal dust from which it came. Thou sendest to man diseases as beneficent messengers to foretell approaching danger and to urge him to avert it.

Thou has blest Thine earth, Thy rivers and Thy mountains with healing substances; they enable Thy creatures to alleviate their sufferings and to heal their illnesses. Thou hast endowed man with the wisdom to relieve the suffering of his brother, to recognize his disorders, to extract the healing substances, to discover their powers and to prepare and to apply them to suit every ill. In Thine Eternal Providence Thou hast chosen me to watch over the life and health of Thy creatures. I am now about to apply myself to the duties of my profession. Support me, Almighty God, in these great labors that they may benefit mankind, for without Thy help not even the least thing will succeed.

Inspire me with love for my art and for Thy creatures. Do not allow thirst for profit, ambition for renown and admiration, to interfere with my profession, for these are the enemies of truth and of love for mankind and they can lead astray in the great task of attending to the welfare of Thy creatures. Preserve the strength of my body and of my soul that they ever be ready to cheerfully help and support rich and poor, good and bad, enemy as well as friend. In the sufferer let me see only the human being. Illumine my mind that it recognize what presents itself and that it may comprehend what is absent or hidden. Let it not fail to see what is visible, but do not permit it to arrogate to itself the power to see what cannot be seen, for delicate and indefinite are the bounds of the great art of caring for the lives and health of Thy creatures. Let me never be absent-minded. May no strange thoughts divert my attention at the bedside of the sick, or disturb my mind in its silent labors, for great and sacred are the thoughtful deliberations required to preserve the lives and health of Thy creatures.

Grant that my patients have confidence in me and my art and follow my directions and my counsel. Remove from their midst all charlatans and the whole host of officious relatives and know-all nurses, cruel people who arrogantly frustrate the wisest purposes of our art and often lead Thy creatures to their death.

Should those who are wiser than I wish to improve and instruct me, let my soul gratefully follow their guidance; for vast is the extent of our art. Should conceited fools, however, censure me, then let love for my profession steel me against them, so that I remain steadfast without regard for age, for reputation, or for honor, because surrender would bring to Thy creatures sickness and death.

Imbue my soul with gentleness and calmness when older colleagues, proud of their age, wish to displace me or to scorn me or disdainfully to teach me. May even this be of advantage to me, for they know many things of which I am ignorant, but let not their arrogance give me pain. For they are old and old age is not master of the passions. I also hope to attain old age upon this earth, before Thee, Almighty God!

Let me be contented in everything except in the great science of my profession. Never allow the thought to arise in me that I have attained to sufficient knowledge, but vouchsafe to me the strength, the leisure and the ambition ever to extend my knowledge. For art is great, but the mind of man is ever expanding.

Almighty God! Thou hast chosen me in Thy mercy to watch over the life and death of Thy creatures. I now apply myself to my profession. Support me in this great task so that it may benefit mankind, for without Thy help not even the least thing will succeed.

### NOTES

1. Luther, *Babylonian Captivity of the Church*, n.p.
2. Luther, *Luther's Works*, 43:129–32.

3. Ibid., 46:252–53.

4. Ibid., 16:344.

5. From E. J. Furcha, ed. and trans., *The Essential Carlstadt: Fifteen Tracts*, 153. Copyright © 1995 Herald Press, Waterloo, Ontario. Used with permission.

6. Calvin, *Institutes of the Christian Religion*, 215–16.

7. Ibid., 273–74.

8. Calvin, *Commentary on a Harmony of the Evangelists*, 250–51.

9. Ibid., 251.

10. Paré, *Journeys in Diverse Places*, 35–36.

11. Paracelsus, *Hermetic and Alchemical Writings*, 203–5.

12. Geoffrey Eatough, *Fracastoro's Syphilis: Introduction, Text, Translation and Notes* (Arca 12) (Liverpool, Great Britain: Francis Cairns, 1984), 101–3. ISBN 978-0-905205-20-5.

13. Burton, *Anatomy of Melancholy*, n.p.

14. "The Handbook of the Militant Christian," from *The Essential Erasmus* by Erasmus, 59–61, trans. John P. Dolan, translation copyright © 1964 by John P. Dolan. Used by permission of New American Library, an imprint of Penguin Publishing Group, a division of Penguin Random House LLC.

15. Teresa of Ávila, *Interior Castle*, 83–84.

16. Ibid., 101–2.

17. Ignatius of Loyola, *Ignatius of Loyola*, 69–71.

18. Ignatius of Loyola, *Spiritual Exercises*, 16.

19. Ignatius of Loyola, *Ignatius of Loyola*, 292.

20. Wesley, *Primitive Physick*, 3–11.

21. From T'ao Lee, "Medical Ethics in Ancient China," *Bulletin of the History of Medicine* 13.1 (1943): 271. Copyright © 1943 The Johns Hopkins Press. Reprinted with permission of Johns Hopkins University Press.

22. Ibid., 274.

23. Friedenwald, "Oath and Prayer of Maimonides," n.p.

# EIGHT

# The Nineteenth through the Twenty-First Centuries

## INTRODUCTION

In this chapter I focus on the intellectual, ethical, and cultural interactions between religion and medicine in the modern era, with particular attention to the twentieth and twenty-first centuries. There has been a vast diversity of modes, particularities, and issues in the intersections between religion and medicine in late modernity across a variety of settings. While it is impossible to fully represent or even briefly sketch this diversity within the limits of a single chapter, I have highlighted texts illustrative of select major themes in the relationship between medicine and religion in this era: religion and contemporary bioethical challenges; spirituality and religion in health care; medicine and new religious movements; global and indigenous religions and medicine; cross-cultural encounters of religions and medicine; religion and global health; and faith healing in the age of science. I have incorporated a broad array of sources representing different geographic, religious, cultural, racial/ethnic, and other contexts. The text selection also reflects the variety of genres and media through which religion has engaged medicine in this era, including travel diaries, letters, liturgies, nonprofit publications, periodicals, professional handbooks, spiritual reflections, ethnographic accounts, theological treatises, conference addresses, autobiographies, and academic monographs.

The modern era introduced new challenges and opportunities into the relationship between religion and medicine. Especially in the West, the unprecedented advancement of biomedical technologies in the second half of the twentieth century raised new questions concerning the ethics of medical interventions and the meaning and boundaries of medical practices.

Traditionally a major source for moral reflection and guidelines, religions became active contributors to these ethical debates. Christianity's long-standing engagement with the question of whether—and to what extent—the use of certain healing and body-altering practices was permissible found expression, among other places, in attempts to articulate Christian principles for accepting or opposing clinical interventions made possible by new technologies.

In the twentieth century, growing secularization in the West eroded many traditional bonds between spiritual care and medical care. However, it did not destroy the recognition that a connection existed between the two. This allowed new forms of integration of both confessional and non-confessional spirituality into health-care practices. Some of the new religious movements that emerged in the nineteenth and twentieth centuries made embracing or rejecting certain medical practices an important part of their identities, at least in popular perception. At the same time, perceived clashes between new scientific and more traditional religious worldviews framed the persistent questions of historical reality and the ongoing occurrence of healing miracles in Christianity in new ways. With a historically unprecedented increase in global migration and transcultural encounters, the cultural uses of health-care practices related to the articulation, preservation, and assertion of minority religious and cultural identities, as well as to the resistance and subversion of the dominant cultures, became more visible. Globalization and pluralism also raised challenges for physicians, who needed to recognize and engage with culturally and religiously specific health-care choices that they might not share or fully understand. Meanwhile, many traditional questions of the history of Christianity and medicine continued into the nineteenth and twentieth centuries. These included the issues of charitable medical service and the ways in which a Christian ethical imperative to self-sacrificially care for weak, vulnerable, and marginalized people could be enacted in the rapidly changing landscape of medical care.

One of the forms through which such Christian charitable impulses found their expression was medical missions. While Catholic missionary activities to the New World developed as early as the sixteenth and seventeenth centuries, the nineteenth century was the heyday of Protestant missionary work in the Global South. With the expansion of Western colonialism in the nineteenth century, the Christianization of native peoples was seen by many Europeans as an integral part of importing Western civilization—which was perceived as superior—to new regions. Medical missionaries could similarly conceive of their work as bringing the knowledge of spiritual salvation through the gospel together with the practical help of Western medicine and the adoption of Western ways of life—all of which were seen as beneficial for native cultures.

An example of such a fusion is the life of David Livingstone, the famed nineteenth-century Scottish missionary to Africa. Livingstone's commitment to promoting "commerce and civilization" alongside Christianity may be better understood in light of his staunch opposition to the African slave trade; he saw the adoption of Western commerce as providing a viable alternative. In his travel diary *Missionary Travels and Researches*, Livingstone recorded how his Christian conversion motivated his desire to study medicine in order to embark on a life of humanitarian service [8.1a]. The diary contained notable anthropological accounts of local religious beliefs about medicine [8.1b].

In the postcolonial world, so-called faith-based organizations conducting community relief work, including medical service, have largely become the new face of Christian charitable missionary endeavors in economically disadvantaged countries of the world. In contrast to certain paternalistic models of Western missions in the colonial era, many of the contemporary nonprofit organizations involved in global health relief efforts tend to work in partnership with local communities, frame their activities more in terms of justice than philanthropy, and stress the inclusive scope of their work. At the same time, they maintain continuity with older ways of conceiving of medical missionary work as grounded in the call of the gospel to self-sacrificially love and serve one's neighbor while maintaining the work's evangelistic dimension, albeit often subsumed under a more primary service orientation. There are tensions between some of these religion-based global health advocates and their secular counterparts over harm reduction programs, such as syringe distribution. Nevertheless, in general, faith-based organizations have proven to be highly effective: in many developing nations, they supply health-care services on an equal level with the countries' respective governments.[1] In its brochure [8.2], World Vision, one of America's largest faith-based relief organizations, with roots in the evangelical Protestant tradition, discusses the benefits of engaging local religious leaders in efforts to improve women's health in Ethiopia.

In 1906, the famous Azusa Street revival began on that eponymous street in Los Angeles, California. This event marked the global emergence of

Pentecostalism, which has its roots in the nineteenth-century holiness movement. Pentecostalism spread rapidly across the world in the twentieth century and altered the landscape of the Christian religion as defined by the more established forms and confessions that grew out of the Protestant Reformation. Pentecostal worshipers remain the fastest-growing segment of Christianity, particularly in parts of the Global South. Along with the trademark practice of glossolalia (speaking in tongues), one of the defining theological aspects of Pentecostalism is an emphasis on the scriptural theme of an all-encompassing struggle between good and evil spiritual forces, and the ongoing reality of miracles, including healing miracles, manifested as part of this warfare. From the very beginning, there was a tradition of a certain degree of suspicion in Pentecostal beliefs regarding human medicine as opposed to direct faith healing. For example, William Seymour, the primary presider over the Azusa Street revival, taught that the use of medicine was only for "unbelievers" [8.3a and b]. One can read this statement as aligned with a marginal Christian tradition seeking to suspend or limit the use of material means in favor of spiritual means, promulgated by such Protestant thinkers as Andreas Carlstadt (see chapter 7).

The Pentecostal emphasis on the continuing occurrence of faith healings in an era characterized by the previously unprecedented capabilities of proof-driven scientific investigations has led to remarkable interactions between scientific study and religious practice. Candy Gunther Brown's ethnographic account of an endeavor to scientifically assess the reality of a supernatural healing incident at a Pentecostal revival meeting in southeastern Africa [8.4] exhibits some of the possibilities and challenges in ongoing encounters between science and religion in our time. The story is also illustrative of current issues in the study of religion and medicine in cross-cultural contexts and of attempts to engage global expressions of Christian healing through Western cultural lenses. "Science at the Crossroads" [8.5] by Tenzin Gyatso, the fourteenth Dalai Lama, highlights the efforts of another global tradition, Tibetan Buddhism, to navigate the complex interactions between religion and contemporary medical science.

A radical conception of matter as irredeemably evil was historically central to the teachings of a number of heterodox religious groups under the general umbrella of Christianity, with so-called Gnostics being one of the earliest examples. In the nineteenth century, such radical philosophical idealism integrated into Christian discourse was promulgated in the writings of Mary Baker Eddy, the founder of a new Christian movement known as Christian Science. Medicine became the special object of Eddy's critique. According to her 1875 *Science and Health with Key to the Scriptures* [8.6], all causes and effects of diseases are mental, not material; and by extension, health is to be understood as a mental rather than a physical condition. She denied the biomedical reality of infections, asserting that infection is the product of a defective human mind, created by an association. Therefore, drugs are superfluous, and "material" medicine is condemned for having originated as an idolatrous practice. Other new religious movements that originated in the nineteenth century, although not denying the material reality of disease, also made health-care issues important to their identity and practice. For example, Jehovah's Witnesses prohibit whole blood transfusions on religious grounds [8.7].

In the twentieth-century West, the development of new, highly sophisticated medical technologies brought about new opportunities for biomedical interventions that had been previously impossible or possible only on a limited scale. These developments generated new ethical questions and provoked intense debates in the public sphere. Where should individuals and society at large draw the boundaries of acceptable biomedical procedures? Should any desired biological intervention altering a human body count as, and be granted the benefits of, a medical procedure? Frequently, references to religion have characterized the rhetoric on all sides of these public debates, contributing to contrasting claims for the moral justification or the denunciation of specific practices. This reality does not mean that all such appeals to religion were equally justifiable, for then religious traditions would be hopelessly confused in their respective moral teachings concerning human life. However, the discernment of the moral position most authentically representing a particular religious tradition in relation to a specific, often historically novel medical practice has proven to be a complicated task, entangled with multiple aspects of ethics and politics.

The late nineteenth and early twentieth centuries saw the rise of an interest in eugenics, a social movement seeking to genetically improve the human race through the prevention of the procreation of "deficient" populations that exhibited possibly hereditary mental, physical, or moral "defects." Eugenics laws prohibiting marriage and even forcing sterilization for certain categories of individuals were adopted in a number of U.S. states and European countries. The response from religious leaders in the West to the moral challenge of eugenics was mixed. In this context Pope Pius XI issued his 1930 encyclical "Casti Connubii" (Of Chaste Marriage) [8.8]. The letter strongly condemned eugenics and the right of the government to forcibly control the marriage and procreation of certain populations deemed "unfit." It also condemned the use of abortion and birth control (although its mention of "natural reasons of time" has been interpreted as support for natural family planning). In the United States, advocacy for contraception (access to which was restricted) at that time was connected to concerns for women's welfare but also often to eugenics goals. Such was the work of Margaret Sanger, a famed American birth-control activist and the founder of what later became the Planned Parenthood Federation of America. Sanger's work focused on the promotion of sex education and contraception as means of improving women's social welfare, empowering women to pursue non-motherhood-related activities, and safeguarding their health by spacing out births and preventing abortions, which Sanger criticized as destroying human lives. At the same time, her advocacy of contraception also supported eugenics practices aimed at decreasing the birth rates of "less desirable" populations. Sanger collaborated with religious leaders and occasionally employed religion in her arguments, as in her 1931 "A Reply to the Pope" [8.9].

Debates about eugenics involving both secular and religious voices assumed a different form in the late twentieth-century West as modifications to human DNA became more feasible. Concerns have been repeatedly voiced that the practice of altering the DNA of select individuals, initially with the noble purpose of exterminating genetic diseases, could eventually lead to the intended or unintended outcome of creating a "superior" human race of genetically enhanced individuals. In the concluding paragraph of his well-known secular work on the subject, *The Future of Human Nature* [8.10], the prominent German philosopher and atheist Jürgen Habermas unexpectedly evoked Judeo-Christian religious traditions in support of his case against "enhancing" genetic modifications of human embryos.

The rapid development of biomedical technologies has forced religious traditions to contextualize their traditional ethics in order to offer moral guidelines with regard to previously unknown or limited biomedical possibilities and specific instances of using contested medical practices. For instance, abortion, although known in premodern eras, became significantly more widespread in the late modern West, partially due to new technologies that made it easier to perform. An example of a religious argument critical of the practice of abortion is Richard Hays's exposition of the ethics expounded in Christian scriptures in his influential work *The Moral Vison of the New Testament* [8.11]. On the opposite side of the debate, the contemporary use of religious practices in abortion-rights advocacy is illustrated by a Unitarian ritual [8.12a] and an interfaith litany in a traditional Christian genre [8.12b] affirming all women's choices as holy, including those for abortion. Similarly, the growing medicalization of death in Western societies has encouraged communities of faith and their leaders to revive some of their respective traditions' spiritual approaches to death and dying. For example, the National Center for Jewish Healing in New York produced a special publication entitled "Jewish Principles of Care for the Dying" [8.14], which offered pathways for the integration of such principles into contemporary medical and North American cultural settings. In a representative illustration from Eastern Orthodox Christianity, John Breck's *The Sacred Gift of Life: Orthodox Christianity and Bioethics* [8.13] brought to light a traditional Eastern Orthodox understanding of a good death, which starkly contrasts with secular Western perspectives. Breck used Orthodox teachings on death to respond to such ethical issues in contemporary medicine as euthanasia and the withdrawal of life support for brain-dead individuals.

In the late modern West, with the dissemination of many traditional cultural forms of religious practice and the growth of self-identified "spiritual but not religious" demographics, the question of the integration of nonsectarian spirituality into medical care gained prominence. The proponents of such integration have tended to emphasize the health and recovery benefits of a patient's spiritual practices or metaphysical beliefs, typically understood as without attachment to traditional religious dogmas or hierarchically prescribed forms of religious thinking. Questions have arisen concerning the lack of defined boundaries for—and therefore the extreme subjectivity of—the notion of the patient's spirituality used in such contexts. If almost any practice or perspective can be understood as expressing an individual's spirituality, should all spiritual practices be equally affirmed, and does the spiritual simply become another tool in the service of the medical? William May's critique [8.15] from a confessional Protestant perspective summarized some of the concerns raised by this approach. At the same time, twentieth-century ethicists continued to probe contemporary answers to the age-old question about the spiritual dimensions of the physician's vocation. In his reflection [8.16], informed by a Catholic intellectual and spiritual tradition, the prominent bioethicist and Franciscan friar Daniel Sulmasy teased out the spiritual aspects of health professionals' everyday work.

A dramatic increase in day-to-day intercultural and interreligious contacts in the twentieth century led to a greater awareness of the multiplicity of ways in which religions and medicine interact in different cultural contexts and the variations in how the connection between the spiritual and the embodied is perceived. In his *Healing with Herbs and Rituals* [8.17], Eliseo Torres described the intertwined material and spiritual dimensions of the traditional Mexican folk healing practices known as *curanderismo*. A glimpse into traditional Native American spiritual practices of healing was provided by Black Elk, a holy man of the Lakota tribe [8.18]. The fusion of the physical and spiritual in African American women's approaches to healing was presented in Stephanie Mitchem's essay [8.19], which revealed the extramedical connotations of the women's quest for well-being. Mohandas Gandhi, in his *Autobiography* [8.20], described dietary and health-care choices as affecting one's character and spirituality.

Increasingly globalized and pluralistic societies have become more aware that a significant misalignment between patients' and physicians' religiously motivated perspectives, expectations, and values with regard to medical treatment compromises the quality of communication and, ultimately, clinical care. I conclude the chapter with two examples of contemporary efforts to make the provision of medical care more responsive to each patient's religious beliefs. In *Patient, Heal Thyself* [8.21], Robert Veatch advocates creating systems of institutional recognition and consideration of patients' beliefs and values in clinical care as essentially underlying all medical decision making. A professional handbook, *Serving the Amish* [8.22], aids health-care workers serving separatist Amish communities in developing a better comprehension of their patients' religious attitudes and practices, equipping them to provide better medical care.

## TEXTS

### 8.1
### Medical missions
David Livingstone, *Missionary Travels and Researches in South Africa*[2]

*David Livingstone (1813–1873) was a Scottish medical missionary, anti-slave-trade activist, and famous geographic explorer of Africa. The passages below are from his immensely popular 1857 book, which combined autobiographical, ethnographic, exploratory, and religious observations from Livingstone's journeys in Africa.*

### a. Conversion to medical service

*This excerpt describes Livingstone's religious motivation in deciding to become a medical missionary (first to China and later to Africa).*

Great pains had been taken by my parents to instill the doctrines of Christianity into my mind, and I had no difficulty in understanding the theory of our free salvation by the atonement of our Savior, but it was only about this time that I really began to feel the necessity and value of a personal application of the provisions of that atonement to my own case. The change was like what may be supposed would take place were it possible to cure a case of "color blindness." The perfect freeness with which the pardon of all our guilt is offered in God's book drew forth feelings of affectionate love to Him who bought us with his blood, and a sense of deep obligation to Him for his mercy has influenced, in some small measure, my conduct ever since. . . .

In the glow of love which Christianity inspires, I soon resolved to devote my life to the alleviation of human misery. Turning this idea over in my mind, I felt that to be a pioneer of Christianity in China might lead to the material benefit of some portions of that immense empire; and therefore set myself to obtain a medical education, in order to be qualified for that enterprise.

### b. Encounters across religions and medicines

*This excerpt is Livingstone's recollection of a cross-cultural encounter between a Western medical doctor and an indigenous "rain doctor" believed to possess religious medicine to cure drought.*

The natives, finding it irksome to sit and wait helplessly until God gives them rain from heaven, entertain the more comfortable idea that they can help themselves by a variety of preparations, such as charcoal made of burned bats, inspissated renal deposit of the mountain cony—"Hyrax capensis"—(which, by the way, is used, in the form of pills, as a good antispasmodic, under the name of "stone-sweat"), the internal parts of different animals—as jackals' livers, baboons' and lions' hearts, and hairy calculi from the bowels of old cows, serpents' skins and vertebrae, and every kind of tuber, bulb, root, and plant to be found in the country. Although you disbelieve their efficacy in charming the clouds to pour out their refreshing treasures, yet, conscious that civility is useful everywhere, you kindly state that you think they are mistaken as to their power. The rain-doctor selects a particular bulbous root, pounds it, and administers a cold infusion to a sheep, which in five minutes afterward expires in convulsions. Part of the same bulb is converted into smoke, and ascends toward the sky; rain follows in a day or two. The inference is obvious. Were we as much harassed by droughts, the logic would be irresistible in England in 1857.

. . .

As for the rain-makers, they carried the sympathies of the people along with them, and not without reason. With the following arguments they were all acquainted, and in order to understand their force, we must place ourselves in their position, and believe, as they do, that all medicines act by a mysterious charm. The term for cure may be translated "charm" ("alaha").

MEDICAL DOCTOR. Hail, friend! How very many medicines you have about you this morning! Why, you have every medicine in the country here.

RAIN DOCTOR. Very true, my friend; and I ought; for the whole country needs the rain which I am making.

M. D. So you really believe that you can command the clouds? I think that can be done by God alone.

R. D. We both believe the very same thing. It is God that makes the rain, but I pray to him by means of these medicines, and, the rain coming, of course it is then mine. It was I who made it for the Bakwains for many years, when they were at Shokuane; through my wisdom, too, their women became fat and shining. Ask them; they will tell you the same as I do.

M. D. But we are distinctly told in the parting words of our Savior that we can pray to God acceptably in his name alone, and not by means of medicines.

R. D. Truly! But God told us differently.

## 8.2
## Religion and global health
World Vision, "Practicing Faith"[3]

*This excerpt is from a brochure produced by the evangelical-founded relief group World Vision, which describes its health-care work in Ethiopia.*

"If we leaders change, the people will follow!"

Those are the words of Tafesse Berhane, a Protestant religious leader in Ethiopia's Guraghe Zone. Berhane's words capture the central message of this book: faith leaders—and communities—have the power to spur far-reaching changes in people's attitudes and behavior. And those changes can bring extraordinary improvements in health and well-being.

The need for change is great. Recent decades have seen improvements on many fronts—on reducing poverty and providing safe drinking water, for example. But when it comes to improving the lives and health of women, change is far too slow in coming.

In Ethiopia—as in many parts of the developing world—women still risk their lives to bring children into the world. Every minute of every day, at least one woman dies from complications related to pregnancy or childbirth—that is some 287,000 every year.

The inequities are stark: A woman in Ethiopia faces a 1 in 50 chance of dying in childbirth; for a woman in Norway, that risk is only about 1 in 15,000. And, for every mother who dies while giving birth, another 20 or 30 survive but sustain life-changing injuries—notably obstetric fistula. Women who suffer from fistula become incontinent, and are often shunned by their communities.

Stunningly, most of these deaths and injuries are completely preventable.

Why, then, do they persist? Women suffer and die because they lack access to prenatal care and skilled birth attendants: only half of women in developing countries receive recommended health care during pregnancy. And they suffer and die because they cannot prevent pregnancies that are unwanted or dangerous.

Sometimes, adequate health services are lacking. Perhaps just as often, services are available, but deep-seated, culturally inscribed beliefs and practices keep women from getting the care they need. Husbands insist that their wives give birth at home, rather than at the health center. Scripture is interpreted in a way that discourages family planning. Harmful traditional practices such as female genital cutting, sometimes referred to as "female circumcision," multiply the dangers of pregnancy and childbirth.

That is where faith leaders come in. Faith leaders possess an unparalleled capacity to shape beliefs and practices. And, in every country on Earth, religious communities are deeply involved in efforts to improve the human condition. In Ethiopia, faith leaders have played a pivotal role in successful responses to health challenges such as HIV/AIDS, and their efforts have helped the Ethiopian government reduce child mortality by half over the last decade.

Today, Ethiopian faith leaders are working with World Vision, government health workers and other partners to improve women's lives and health.

## 8.3
## Faith healing: Pentecostalism

*These excerpts are from the periodical* Apostolic Faith, *in which the Azusa Street Mission used to offer theological guidance to the Pentecostal movement.*

### a. Revival of faith healings
Azusa Street Mission, *Apostolic Faith*[4]

The Lord is graciously healing many sick bodies. People are healed at the Mission almost every day. Requests come in for prayer from all over. They are presented in the meeting and the Spirit witnesses in many cases that prayer is answered, and when we hear from them they are healed. Handkerchiefs are sent to be blest, and are returned to the sick and they are healed in many cases. One day nine handkerchiefs were blest, another day sixteen. A man came with a broken arm and was healed. The mission people never take medicine. They do not want it. They have taken Jesus for their healer and He always heals.

. . .

Sickness is all the work of Satan. Sometimes we bring it upon ourselves by overexertion. Sometimes it is permitted of the Lord because of sins of omission or commission. Satan cannot afflict us unless God permits. He has no power over us unless we get on his territory.

## b. *"Medicine is for unbelievers"*
Azusa Street Mission, *Apostolic Faith*[5]

Do you teach that it is wrong to take medicine?

Yes, for saints to take medicine. Medicine is for unbelievers, but the remedy for the saints of God we will find in James 5:14, "Is any sick among you, let him call for the elders of the church, and let them pray over him, anointing him with oil in the name of the Lord, and the prayer of faith shall save the sick, and the Lord shall raise him up; and if he have committed sins, they shall be forgiven him."

. . .

Does the Lord Jesus provide healing for everybody?

Yes; for all those who have faith in Him. The sinner can receive healing.

### 8.4
### Science and world religions I: Global Christianity
Candy Gunther Brown, *Testing Prayer*[6]

*This excerpt records a healing ritual performed by a traveling evangelist in rural Mozambique.*

Preaching from a makeshift bamboo platform in a typical mud-hut village in northern Mozambique, near the southeast coast of Africa, Heidi Baker issued a *promessa*, or promise: "Bring me your deaf, and Jesus will heal them, in confirmation of the truth of the gospel." The moon was almost full on this clear, tropical winter night. In the comfortable 80-degree weather, most of the thousand-person, predominantly Muslim village had come out. They were attracted by the showing of the *Jesus Film*, in the local Makua language, on a portable projector and screen with the help of generator-powered stage lights and a booming sound system. "Bring me your deaf!" Mama Aida, as Baker had come to be known, repeated in ringing tones in both Portuguese and Makua. A young adult man, Jordan, was soon brought by his father and a quickly gathering crowd of villagers, all of whom chimed that Jordan had been deaf and mute since birth. Before Baker prayed for him, on this particular evening she had given permission for a western research group to test his hearing, using a portable audiometry machine that administered tones of increasing intensities through headphones. The audiometer produced tones all the way up to 100 decibels hearing level (dBHL) in each ear—louder than a motorcycle—but there was still no response by the subject. Using gestures, Jordan replied negatively to his father's query as to whether he had heard anything.

Baker put her arms around Jordan and prayed for less than a minute, commanding his ears to be opened in Jesus's name. She then asked Jordan to repeat after her as she spoke from behind his line of sight: "Jezush," "Hallelujah," and clapped her hands and snapped her fingers at increasing distances. Jordan imitated the words in a hoarse, raspy voice, and clapped and snapped after Baker, to the apparent amazement of the crowd, who insisted that he had never before heard or spoken at all. My research group reinstalled the headphones and tried to explain to the subject how to press the audiometer's response button as soon as he heard a tone. Jordan pressed the response button when some of the tones reached 60 dBHL (0 dBHL being perfect hearing)—not terrible, given that the ambient noise from the commotion of the crowd and the still-playing sound system remained around 80 decibels sound pressure level (dBSPL). But unless the subject was constantly reminded to press the button when he heard a tone, he apparently forgot the instructions in the excitement of new sensory input and an interested crowd of villagers, missionaries, and researchers all focusing their attention on him. Jordan seemed to press the button consistently whenever we reminded him that he should press the button when he heard a sound, but otherwise he did not press the button. He responded more reliably when instead asked to imitate the tone when he heard it, or when asked after each tone (or nontone, silences that tested for false-positive responses) whether he had heard anything.

Explaining how to take a hearing test in the context of an illiterate culture to someone apparently unaccustomed to the communication of complex ideas seemed to present more of a challenge than the researchers had anticipated. Alternatively, Jordan's hearing had not improved, but he only appeared to respond to tones because he coincidentally pressed the button or made sounds when tones were being administered. In either case, the audiometer repeatedly aborted its automated protocol due to inconsistent responses. After switching to the manual mode and getting a few false positives mixed in with some consistent responses, we finally gave up after forty-five minutes of trying to measure the subject's hearing, and excluded the results from the analysis. Nevertheless, it seemed obvious to everyone present that Jordan was repeating sounds in his environment, whereas a few minutes before he had appeared oblivious even to very loud noise. At the platform, Baker gave an altar call for "salvation from sin," and a number of people in the crowd responded. The following morning, two Muslim men sought out the small village church, wanting to convert to Christianity because they had heard about the apparent miracle. Did Baker's prayers result in a cure of deafness, and was it "miraculous"? How can scholars account for this apparent success of healing prayer—despite the failure of western technology to measure it?

## 8.5
### Science and world religions II: Buddhism
Tenzin Gyatso, "Science at the Crossroads"[7]

*The following excerpt is from the fourteenth Dalai Lama's address at a Society for Neuroscience meeting in Washington, DC.*

Since the primary motive underlying the Buddhist investigation of reality is the fundamental quest for overcoming suffering and perfecting the human condition, the primary orientation of the Buddhist investigative tradition has been toward understanding the human mind and its various functions. The assumption here is that by gaining deeper insight into the human psyche, we might find ways of transforming our thoughts, emotions and their underlying propensities so that a more wholesome and fulfilling way of being can be found. It is in this context that the Buddhist tradition has devised a rich classification of mental states, as well as contemplative techniques for refining specific mental qualities. So a genuine exchange between the cumulative knowledge and experience of Buddhism and modern science on wide-ranging issues pertaining to the human mind, from cognition and emotion to understanding the capacity for transformation inherent in the human brain can be deeply interesting and potentially beneficial as well. In my own experience, I have felt deeply enriched by engaging in conversations with neuroscientists and psychologists on such questions as the nature and role of positive and negative emotions, attention, imagery, as well {as} the plasticity of the brain. The compelling evidence from neuroscience and medical science of the crucial role of simple physical touch for even the physical enlargement of an infant's brain during the first few weeks powerfully brings home the intimate connection between compassion and human happiness.

Buddhism has long argued for the tremendous potential for transformation that exists naturally in the human mind. To this end, the tradition has developed a wide range of contemplative techniques, or meditation practices, aimed specifically at two principal objectives—the cultivation of a compassionate heart and the cultivation of deep insights into the nature of reality, which are referred to as the union of compassion and wisdom. At the heart of these meditation practices lie two key techniques, the refinement of attention and its sustained application on the one hand, and the regulation and transformation of emotions on the other. In both of these cases, I feel, there might be great potential for collaborative research between the Buddhist contemplative tradition and neuroscience.

## 8.6
### New religious movements I: Christian Science
Mary Baker Eddy, *Science and Health with Key to the Scriptures*[8]

*This excerpt is from the foundational work of the Church of Christ, Scientist, established by Mary Baker Eddy (1821–1910).*

Jesus never spoke of disease as dangerous or as difficult to heal. When his students brought to him a case they had failed to heal, he said to them, "O faithless generation," implying that the requisite power to heal was in Mind. He prescribed no drugs, urged no obedience to material laws, but acted in direct disobedience to them. . . .

Disease arises, like other mental conditions, from association. Since it is a law of mortal mind that certain diseases should be regarded as contagious, this law obtains credit through association,—calling up the fear that creates the image of disease and its consequent manifestation in the body. . . .

Christian Science exterminates the drug, and rests on Mind alone as the curative Principle, acknowledging that the divine Mind has all power. . . .

If drugs are part of God's creation, which (according to the narrative in Genesis) He pronounced *good*, then drugs cannot be poisonous. If He could create drugs intrinsically bad, then they should never be used. If He creates drugs at all and designs them for medical use, why did Jesus not employ them and recommend them for the treatment of disease? Matter is not self-creative, for it is unintelligent. Erring mortal mind confers the power which the drug seems to possess.

Narcotics quiet mortal mind, and so relieve the body; but they leave both mind and body worse for this submission. Christian Science impresses the entire corporeality,—namely, mind and body,—and brings out the proof that Life is continuous and harmonious. Science both neutralizes error and destroys it. Mankind is the better for this spiritual and profound pathology.

It is recorded that the profession of medicine originated in idolatry with pagan priests, who besought the gods to heal the sick and designated Apollo as "the god of medicine." He was supposed to have dictated the first prescription, according to the "History of Four Thousand Years of Medicine." It is here noticeable that Apollo was also regarded as the sender of disease, "the god of pestilence." Hippocrates turned from image-gods to vegetable and mineral drugs for healing. This was deemed progress in medicine; but what we need is the truth which heals both mind and body. The future history of material medicine may correspond with that of its material god, Apollo, who was banished from heaven and endured great sufferings upon earth.

Drugs, cataplasms, and whiskey are stupid substitutes for the dignity and potency of divine Mind and its efficacy to heal. It is pitiful to lead men into temptation through the byways of this wilderness world,—to victimize the race with intoxicating prescriptions for the sick, until mortal mind acquires an educated appetite for strong drink, and men and women become loathsome sots. . . .

The medical schools would learn the state of man from matter instead of from Mind. They examine the lungs, tongue, and pulse to ascertain how much harmony, or health, matter is permitting to matter,—how much pain or pleasure, action or stagnation, one form of matter is allowing another form of matter.

Ignorant of the fact that a man's belief produces disease and all its symptoms, the ordinary physician is liable to increase disease with his own mind, when he should address himself to the work of destroying it through the power of the divine Mind. . . .

The ordinary practitioner, examining bodily symptoms, telling the patient that he is sick, and treating the case according to his physical diagnosis, would naturally induce the very disease he is trying to cure, even if it were not already determined by mortal mind. Such unconscious mistakes would not occur, if this old class of philanthropists looked as deeply for cause and effect into mind as into matter. The physician agrees with his "adversary quickly," but upon different terms than does the metaphysician;

for the matter-physician agrees with the disease, while the metaphysician agrees only with health and challenges disease.

Christian Science brings to the body the sunlight of Truth, which invigorates and purifies. Christian Science acts as an alternative, neutralizing error with Truth. It changes the secretions, expels humors, dissolves tumors, relaxes rigid muscles, restores carious bones to soundness. The effect of this Science is to stir the human mind to a change of base, on which it may yield to the harmony of the divine Mind.

## 8.7
## New religious movements II: Jehovah's Witnesses
"What Does the Bible Say About Blood Transfusions?"[9]

*This statement outlines the Jehovah's Witnesses' religious rationale behind the prohibition of whole blood transfusions. The explanation is based on interpreting select Old Testament passages that forbid the consumption of blood as applicable to the receiving of blood for medical purposes.*

The Bible commands that we not ingest blood. So we should not accept whole blood or its primary components in any form, whether offered as food or as a transfusion. Note the following scriptures:

Genesis 9:4. God allowed Noah and his family to add animal flesh to their diet after the Flood but commanded them not to eat the blood. God told Noah: "Only flesh with its soul—its blood—you must not eat." This command applies to all mankind from that time on because all are descendants of Noah.

Leviticus 17:14. "You must not eat the blood of any sort of flesh, because the soul of every sort of flesh is its blood. Anyone eating it will be cut off." God viewed the soul, or life, as being in the blood and belonging to him. Although this law was given only to the nation of Israel, it shows how seriously God viewed the law against eating blood.

Acts 15:20. "Abstain . . . from blood." God gave Christians the same command that he had given to Noah. History shows that early Christians refused to consume whole blood or even to use it for medical reasons.

Why does God command us to abstain from blood? There are sound medical reasons to avoid blood transfusions. More important, though, God commands that we abstain from blood because what it represents is sacred to him.

## 8.8
### Religion and bioethical polemics I: Contraception and eugenics
Pope Pius XI, "Casti Connubii"[10]

*These excerpts are from a 1930 encyclical, an official papal letter to Roman Catholic bishops, written by Pope Pius XI (1857–1939) and entitled "Casti Connubii" (Of Chaste Marriage). Parts 10–13 formulated a theology of marriage as largely oriented around human procreation, which served as a justification for the denunciation of contraception in part 56. Parts 68–69 condemned eugenics and specifically the eugenics laws of the era, which made it illegal for certain "defective" populations to marry and have children.*

10. Now when We come to explain, Venerable Brethren, what are the blessings that God has attached to true matrimony, and how great they are, there occur to Us the words of that illustrious Doctor of the Church whom We commemorated recently in Our Encyclical *Ad salutem* on the occasion of the fifteenth centenary of his death [Encycl. *Ad salutem*, 20 April 1930]: "These," says St. Augustine, "are all the blessings of matrimony on account of which matrimony itself is a blessing; offspring, conjugal faith and the sacrament" [St. August., *De bono coniug.*, cap. 24, n. 32]. . . .

11. Thus amongst the blessings of marriage, the child holds the first place. And indeed the Creator of the human race Himself, Who in His goodness wishes to use men as His helpers in the propagation of life, taught this when, instituting marriage in Paradise, He said to our first parents, and through them to all future spouses: "Increase and multiply, and fill the earth" [*Gen.*, I, 28]. As St. Augustine admirably deduces from the words of the holy Apostle Saint Paul to Timothy [*I Tim.*, V, 14] when he says: "The Apostle himself is therefore a witness that marriage is for the sake of generation: 'I wish,' he says, 'young girls to marry.' And, as if someone said to him, 'Why?,' he immediately adds: 'To bear children, to be mothers of families' " [St. August., *De bono coniug.*, cap. 24, n. 32].

. . .

13. But Christian parents must also understand that they are destined not only to propagate and preserve the human race on earth, indeed not only to educate any kind of worshippers of the true God, but children who are to become members of the Church of Christ, to raise up fellow-citizens of the Saints, and members of God's household [*Eph.*, II, 19], that the worshippers of God and Our Savior may daily increase.

. . .

56. Since, therefore, openly departing from the uninterrupted Christian tradition some recently have judged it possible solemnly to declare another doctrine regarding this question, the Catholic Church, to whom God has entrusted the defense of the integrity and purity of morals, standing erect in the midst of the moral ruin which surrounds her, in order that she may preserve the chastity of the nuptial union from being defiled by this foul stain, raises her voice in token of her divine ambassadorship and through Our mouth proclaims anew: any use whatsoever of matrimony exercised in such a way that the act is deliberately frustrated in its natural power to generate life is an offense against the law of God and of nature, and those who indulge in such are branded with the guilt of a grave sin.

. . .

68. Finally, that pernicious practice must be condemned which closely touches upon the natural right of man to enter matrimony but affects also in a real way the welfare of the offspring. For there are some who over solicitous for the cause of eugenics, not only give salutary counsel for more certainly procuring the strength and health of the future child—which, indeed, is not contrary to right reason—but put eugenics before aims of a higher order, and by public authority wish to prevent from marrying all those whom, even though naturally fit for marriage, they consider, according to the norms and conjectures of their investigations, would, through hereditary transmission, bring forth defective offspring. And more, they wish to legislate to deprive these of that natural faculty by medical action despite their unwillingness; and this they do not propose as an infliction of grave punishment under the authority of the state for a crime committed, not to prevent future crimes by guilty persons, but against every right and good they wish the civil authority to arrogate to itself a power over a faculty which it never had and can never legitimately possess.

69. Those who act in this way are at fault in losing sight of the fact that the family is more sacred than the State and that men are begotten not for the earth and for time, but for Heaven and eternity. Although often these individuals are to be dissuaded from entering into matrimony, certainly it is wrong to brand men with the stigma of crime because they contract marriage, on the ground that, despite the fact that they are in every respect capable of matrimony, they will give birth only to defective children, even though they use all care and diligence.

### 8.9
## Religion and bioethical polemics II: An opposing perspective
Margaret Sanger, "Birth Control Advances: A Reply to the Pope"[11]

*This essay, written in 1931, was a response by Margaret Sanger (1879–1966) to Pope Pius XI's 1930 encyclical "Casti Connubii." Sanger attacked the pope's argument that childbearing is the chief goal of marriage as misguided and no longer relevant. She also outlined socioeconomic, health, and religious reasons for birth control, including eugenics, by implying that God is concerned with the life-span as well as the "quality" versus "quantity" of people.*

The steady advance of the birth control movement can only receive fresh impetus from the new interest which has been aroused by the attack of Pope Pius XI.

His encyclical letter, "Of Chaste Marriage," made public in January, 1931, aims to regulate the conjugal affairs of Catholic men and women, without the benefit of science, and according to theories written by St. Augustine, also a bachelor, who died fifteen centuries ago. The Pope makes it perfectly plain that Catholics are expected to give up health, happiness, and life itself while making every other conceivable sacrifice rather than to have dominion over nature's processes of procreation. His letter denies that any claims of poverty, sickness, or other hindrances to proper rearing of children are valid reasons for the scientific limitation of offspring. As for the breeding of criminal, diseased, feeble-minded, and insane classes, the Pope opposes every method of control except that of suggesting to these unfortunate people to please not do it any more.

One must deplore the fact that Pope Pius should have chosen this time of the world's distress from unemployment, poverty, and economic maladjustment to advertise doctrines and advise conduct which can only tend to aggravate that distress. . . .

Now comes the question of how many children there should be in a family. There is a Biblical story of how God told the creatures of the sea to "increase and multiply and fill the waters," and how He told Adam and Eve to "increase and multiply and fill the earth." The population movement which then started got a terrific setback in God's Great Flood, but we are told that He gave exactly the same command to Noah and his family group—"Increase and multiply and fill the earth." The Pope quotes the Adam and Eve part of this story together with the endorsement of the good St. Augustine, who died a thousand years before America was discovered. It strikes me that St. Augustine, however, is not a true believer in the doctrine, for I understand that he had only one son (illegitimate) and that he said, "No fruitfulness of the flesh can be compared to holy virginity." The Pope declares further:

"But Christian parents must also understand that they are destined not only to propagate and preserve the human race on earth, indeed not only to educate any kind of worshipers of the true God, but children who are to become members of the Church of Christ, to raise up fellow-citizens of the saints and members of God's household, that the worshippers of God and our Savior may daily increase."

Repeating these two points in everyday language, the Pope commands married women to bear numerous children, a. To fill the earth, and, b. To increase the membership in the Catholic Church.

Assuming for the sake of argument that God does want an increasing number of worshippers of the Catholic faith, does he want the throng to include an increasing number of feeble-minded, insane, criminal, and diseased worshipers? That is unavoidable, if the Pope is obeyed, because he forbids every single method of birth control except continence, a method which the feeble-minded, insane and criminal people will not use.

If God is interested in numbers rather than in quality of people, if He wants what business men call a "rapid turnover," and if he prefers children to adults in the Heavenly choir of praise, then indiscriminate breeding of human beings is indicated. It is a well-known fact that those races or groups of people which have the greatest number of births per mother also have the greatest infant mortality. And as for the character of those who survive, remember what Jesus said in the Sermon on the Mount, "Do men gather grapes of thorns or figs of thistles? A corrupt tree cannot bring forth good fruit."

## 8.10

## Religion and new technologies: DNA enhancement

Jürgen Habermas, *The Future of Human Nature*[12]

*This excerpt is from the concluding paragraphs of the contemporary German philosopher Jürgen Habermas's otherwise secular case against "enhancing" genetic modifications of human embryos. At the core of Habermas's argument lies the assertion that modifications of an embryo's DNA at the request of others would radically undermine the most basic grounds of human equality and freedom. Such a loss of equality will occur if individuals are allowed to assume the role of each other's creators and intentionally design other people according to their specific likings.*

In the controversy, for instance, about the way to deal with human embryos, many voices still evoke the first book of Moses, Genesis 1:27: "So God created man in his own image, in the image of God created he him." In order to understand what *Gottesebenbildlichkeit*—"in the likeness of God"—means, one need not believe that the God who is love creates, with Adam and Eve, free creatures who are like him. One knows that there can be no love without recognition of the self in the other, nor freedom without mutual recognition. So, the other who has human form must himself be free in order to be able to return God's affection. In spite of his likeness to God, however, this other is also imagined as being God's creature. Regarding his origin, he cannot be of equal birth with God. This *creatural nature* of the image expresses an intuition which in the present context may even speak to those who are tone-deaf to religious connotations. . . .

Because he is both in one, God the Creator and God the Redeemer, this creator does not need, in his actions, to abide by the laws of nature like a technician, or by the rules of a code like a biologist or computer scientist. From the very beginning, the voice of God calling into life communicates within a morally sensitive universe. Therefore God may "determine" man in the sense of enabling and, at the same time, obliging him to be free. Now, one need not believe in theological premises in order to understand what follows from this, namely, that an entirely different kind of dependence, perceived as a causal one, becomes involved if the difference assumed as inherent in the concept of creation were to disappear, and the place of God be taken by a peer—if, that is, a human being would intervene, according to his own preferences and without being justified in assuming, at least counterfactually, a consent of the concerned other, in the random combination of the parents' sets of chromosomes. This reading leads to the question I have dealt with elsewhere: Would not the first human being to determine, *at his own discretion*, the natural essence of another human being at the same time destroy the equal freedoms that exist among persons of equal birth in order to ensure their difference?

## 8.11
## Religion and bioethical polemics III: Abortion
Richard Hays, *The Moral Vision of the New Testament*[13]

*In this passage, a United Methodist New Testament scholar, Richard Hays, provided a religious perspective on a central question of nonsectarian bioethical debates about abortion: whether human embryos and fetuses should be considered human "persons" worthy of a protected status like members of the human species at other stages of development. He analyzed Luke 10:25–37, according to which an expert in Jewish religious law, in light of its key commandment to love one's neighbor as oneself, posed the question "Who is my neighbor?" In response, Jesus told a parable that extended the category of a neighbor (assumed to refer to a fellow Israelite) to a merciful Samaritan, a despised outsider.*

Jesus' parable {of the good Samaritan; Luke 10:25–37} offers a category-shattering answer to the question, "Who is my neighbor?" The double love command, citing Deuteronomy 6:5 and Leviticus 19:18, enjoins love of God and of neighbor (10:27), but the lawyer presses for a more precise delineation of the term "neighbor"—which in the original context of Leviticus meant "fellow Israelite." Jesus' story about the compassionate Samaritan, however, rather than narrowing down the definition of "neighbor," reshapes the whole issue in two ways: the hated Samaritan becomes included in the category of "neighbor," and the "neighbor" is defined as one who *shows* rather than *receives*, mercy (10:36–37).

How does this story illuminate the issue of abortion? The point is not that the unborn child is by definition a "neighbor." Rather, the point is that we are called upon to *become* neighbors to those who are helpless, going beyond conventional conceptions of duty to provide life-sustaining aid to those whom we might not have regarded as worthy of our compassion. Such a standard would apply both to the mother in a "crisis pregnancy" and to her unborn child. When we ask, "Is the fetus a person?" we are asking the same sort of limiting, self-justifying question that the lawyer asked Jesus: "Who is my neighbor?" *Jesus, by answering the lawyer's question with this parable, rejects casuistic attempts to circumscribe our moral concern by defining the other as belonging to a category outside the scope of our obligation.* To define the unborn child as a nonperson is to narrow the scope of moral concern, whereas Jesus calls upon us to widen it by show-ing mercy and actively intervening on behalf of the helpless. The Samari-tan is a paradigm of love that goes beyond ordinary obligation and thus *creates* a neighbor relation where none existed before. The concluding word of the parable addresses us all: "Go and do likewise." What would it mean for our decisions about abortion if we did indeed take the Samaritan as a paradigm?

**8.12**

**Religion and bioethical polemics IV: An opposing perspective**

*The passages below illustrate the use of religious rituals in support of and in current advocacy for abortion rights. The resources were provided by the Reli-gious Coalition for Reproductive Choice, an advocacy group working with rep-resentatives from various religious traditions to morally and legally defend unrestricted access to abortion.*

### *a. Ceremony for closure after an abortion*
Religious Coalition for Reproductive Choice, *Prayerfully Pro-Choice: Resources for Worship*[14]

*This religious ritual is in the Unitarian Universalist tradition.*

(Spoken by the minister)
We use the petals of a budding rose as a symbol of all the potential which might have been incarnated in _____ and _____'s child. With loving grief, we release that potential to other incarnations in the infinite womb of the universe, from which nothing is ever lost.

(The minister breaks the petals from the stem of the rose, and gives them to the couple to hold. Then the minister says:)

However gently, the bud is broken.
In pain and sorrow the Word is spoken:
Not every essence shall come to be;
It is in choosing that we are free.

(The couple scatters the petals on the water in the bowl.)

## b. *Diann L. Neu,* A Litany of Challenge

Religious Coalition for Reproductive Choice, *Prayerfully Pro-Choice: Resources for Worship*[15]

*This interfaith liturgy employs the traditional Christian genre of litany.*

All: Let us go forth.

Leader: To stand, sit, cry, pray, with women making reproductive choices, especially the difficult choice for abortion.

All: Let us go forth.

Leader: To speak to legislators, family members and friends of our support for women's decisions.

All: Let us go forth.

Leader: To challenge our synagogues, churches and holy congregations to affirm women as moral agents.

All: Let us go forth.

Leader: To encourage rabbis, ministers, priests and counselors to counsel women on free choice.

All: Let us go forth.

Leader: To the city centers and country corners to tell women that all of their choices, including their choice for abortion, are holy and healthy.

All: Let us go forth.

Leader: In the name of the holy one, God of our mothers and God of our fathers, to bring about justice.

## 8.13

## New issues in end-of-life care I: Eastern Orthodox Christianity

John Breck, *The Sacred Gift of Life*[16]

*This text by Father John Breck uses traditional Eastern Orthodox teachings about a good death to respond to contemporary bioethical controversies surrounding the ethics of ending a life.*

The Park Ridge Center publication *Choosing Death* includes several statements by Orthodox ethicists on the matter of active euthanasia, the intentional medical termination of a human life. They reflect a consensus that has emerged in recent years and can be summarized as follows. 1) Human life, created by God and bearing the divine image, is sacred by its very nature and must always be respected and protected as such. 2) The principle of stewardship demands that the moment of death, like that of conception, remain in the hands of God; he alone is sovereign over life, death and the dying process. There is "a time to live and a time to die," and that time must remain in God's determination. 3) Every effort must be made to restore the patient to an optimal state of health; the patient's life, however, retains its irreducible value and worth, even when full health cannot be restored. 4) In cases of terminal illness (where the dying process is irreversible and death is imminent), it is nevertheless permissible to withhold or withdraw life-support that represents nothing more than a burden to the patient. Particularly in cases of brain-death, it is immoral—and not merely "useless"—to maintain the patient on life-support systems. 5) On the other hand, there can be no justification for the active taking of (innocent) human life, even in cases of terminal illness accompanied by severe suffering. Active euthanasia, including physician-assisted suicide, is therefore forbidden by an Orthodox ethic, whether or not the patient expresses the desire to die, that is, whether or not there is informed consent.

. . .

Traditional Orthodox piety expresses the desire to be spared from "a sudden death." To most Americans today, such a request is incomprehensible: "Let it be swift, clean, and if possible, in my sleep . . ." A genuinely Christian attitude, on the other hand, recognizes the need to prepare for death: to allow time for the dying patient to seek reconciliation and fellowship with family members and friends, time to seek reconciliation with God through confession, and time for a final communion in the life-giving Body and Blood of Christ. This need to prepare for the end of earthly existence is what explains the frequency of prayers in the Orthodox tradition that implore God, "Lord, spare me from an unexpected death!" To "die well," then, requires *time* as much as it requires inner peace, appropriate care, and love.

## 8.14
### New issues in end-of-life care II: Judaism
National Center for Jewish Healing, "Jewish Principles
of Care for the Dying"[17]

*The excerpt is from a special 2001 edition of the National Center for Jewish Healing's newsletter, the* Outstretched Arm, *published from 1991 to 2010. The center, a part of the Jewish healing movement, worked to revive ancient and to produce new Jewish spiritual approaches to healing in the context of the contemporary North American health-care landscape. The passage was adapted from Rabbi Amy Eilberg's "Acts of Loving Kindness: A Training Manual for Bikur Holim."*

Here are some Jewish principles of care for the dying which are helpful to keep in mind:

### B'tselem Elohim (created in the image of the Divine):

This is true no matter what the circumstances at the final stage of life. Often it is our task to simply see that no matter how much time remains until the moment of death, this person embodies a spark of the Divine.

### Refu'at HaNefesh (healing of the spirit):

With surprising frequency, the final stages of life offer the possibility of healing of the spirit, precisely when healing of the body is no longer a possibility. It is helpful to simply know this truth, and perhaps to remember occasions when one has seen this in life.

### Hopefulness:

As long as there is life, there is hope. It is not helpful to encourage unrealistic expectations on the level of physical healing, lest the patient and loved ones feel betrayed and shattered when this hope proves unjustified. There are things to hope for, and an attitude of hopefulness is possible even in dark times.

### Teshuva (repentance/turning/atonement):

One Talmudic rabbi taught, "Do *teshuva* the day before you die." This poignant teaching encourages all of us to live our lives in such a way that we will be ready when death comes. It helps to know that extraordinary acts of soul-searching, reconciliation, and growth can and do happen right up to the end of life.

### Community:

Inevitably, we die alone, in our own body, on our own solitary journey. Yet as with every phase of the Jew's life, we journey with others, those who have gone before and those who stand with us now. We are part of this larger community (a Jewish community, a human community) that has known death and will continue to live after our bodies are gone—part of something stronger and larger than death.

**Appreciation of everyday miracles:**

Quite often, the nearness of death awakens a powerful appreciation of the "miracles that are with us, morning, noon and night" (in the language of the Amidah prayer). Appreciation loves company; we only need to say "yes" when people express these things.

### 8.15
### Spirituality in health care I: Protestantism
William May, *The Physician's Covenant*[18]

*This passage by the medical ethicist William May presented a mainline Presbyterian Christian critique of some dimensions of nonsectarian advocacy for a positive role of spirituality in health care, which May viewed as ultimately instrumentalizing the transcendent.*

My chief objection to the current literature on religion and health is religious rather than empirical or moral. The literature sometimes caters to a narcissism in the believer and thus runs the risk of instrumentalizing and therefore trivializing God. First, too much of the literature on the role of religion in healing focuses too narrowly on the afflicted believer and his or her immediate circle of family and friends. In medical crisis, Scripture certainly authorizes believers to pray and to intercede for help: "Father, let this cup pass from me . . ." But the afflicted and their company of relatives and friends should also pray within a discipline that pares away all narcissism—"nevertheless, not my will but thine be done." A narrow focus on one's own plight can overlook the broader reach of intercessory prayer as it extends beyond one's circle of intimates toward the stranger and the forlorn. Such prayer implies a wider religious responsibility for health care. The church spaciously acts on the full scope of intercessory prayer when, in addition to specific prayers for healing, it also founds and supports hospitals; inspires doctors, nurses, social workers, and chaplains vocationally; develops institutions such as hospices, drug addiction programs, and medical self-help organizations; and tackles social problems such as hunger, poverty, and housing, which bear on the health of citizens.

Further, to justify religious belief and practice simply on the grounds that they improve one's health and lengthen one's life can convert God into a spiritual tool in the shed. Some secondary health benefits (and moral benefits) accrue from worship, but we hardly know what we are doing in worship if we worship God for that reason alone. The Supreme Being is an end in itself, not the means to some other end. Married people tend to live longer than single people. But we would question John's motives for marrying Jane if he married her on the grounds that marriage would yield him some extra months or years of life. Jane might reasonably think of herself as used rather than loved.

The love of God, rightly understood, lifts us out of the instrumental realm of "so that" and "in order to." Worship places us before the "I am that I am." To worship God "in order to" lower one's blood pressure, earn more money, catch an extra hour's sleep, or lengthen one's life confuses creaturely goods with the deity.

## 8.16
## Spirituality in health care II: Catholicism
### Daniel Sulmasy, *A Balm for Gilead*[19]

*In the following passage informed by the Roman Catholic spiritual tradition, the medical ethicist, physician, and Franciscan friar Daniel Sulmasy called fellow medical professionals to the cultivation of personal devotional practices as a foundation for their healing work. By analyzing a physician's response to a simple case of a skin infection in a young woman, Sulmasy drew attention to the presence of the transcendent in what may appear to be a mundane clinical encounter.*

The rhythm of prayer and healing that informed the public life of Jesus Christ forms the perfect pattern for the Christian healer to emulate. Prayer is the opening of one's whole self to God. Between the "peak" experiences of the numinous, one must translate those experiences into daily life—at work and at home. One must continue to cultivate one's spirit, to let God speak not just on the mountaintop but also in the public square. In the public square of medicine, God tugs at the hem of one's white coat and asks for healing. One must cultivate the ability to sense when power goes out from one's own body and others are healed (Lk 8:46). Most clinicians remain blithely unaware.

To heal is to restore the state of right relations in a whole person. A healer whose own relations are set right is naturally in a better position to heal. One starts with one's own spirituality, one's own relationship with the transcendent, one's own experience of the Numinous One. To be an effective healer requires the true self-knowledge that comes only from a spiritual source. "What a person is before God, that he is, and no more," say the Admonitions of St. Francis. . . . Once one knows who one is in relationship to God, all other relationships fall more easily into place, including one's relationships with patients.

The ways one can accomplish this self-knowledge, even in the busy life of a clinician, are actually many and varied. One may prefer journaling, centering prayer, the rosary, Christian yogic meditation, *lectio divina* (a slow, contemplative method of reading scripture), or something else. The exact method is less important than the committed, intentional act. Busy people might also benefit by learning to become "opportunistic" pray-ers. What I mean by this is that one can take advantage of situations such as commuting (whether by public transportation or personal automobile) and learn to turn the delays and breakdowns into moments of prayer. Traffic jams can be transformed into graced moments with God rather than occasions of road rage. One need not spend all one's commuting time listening to Continuing Medical Education tapes. Dictating office notes while driving can be dangerous. Why not pray instead?

Although God can certainly appear when least expected, one can commit oneself to habitual practices of prayer that predispose one to hearing God's voice. One can prayerfully remember patients at the end of the day or cultivate a reverent mindfulness in one's daily practice. But whatever way one prays, it is important that one's practice inform one's spirituality every bit as much as one's spirituality ought to inform one's practice. That is the rhythm of Christian contemplation and action.

The transcendent questions of meaning, value, and relationship that are the fundamental questions of spirituality are visible everywhere in one's practice—provided one's eyes have been opened, and one has learned how to see. The transcendent can be found in the simple and the mundane.

For example, a twenty-four-year-old graduate student may show up as a walk-in to the office with a chief complaint of a new spot on her skin. She might say, "I've got this spot. It's been growing. Yesterday a friend saw it and said it looked like ringworm. I said it couldn't be ringworm. I mean, I take a bath every day. I'm a clean person."

One's temptation as a clinician is to the supercilious—to delight in one's superior knowledge and in the patient's ignorance. The physician knows this is not a hygiene problem. But the patient was truly troubled, in a simple way, by the *meaning* of what had befallen her. She was asking, indirectly, "Does this mean I'm dirty?"

She was also presenting with genuine questions of value: "What must people think of me now that I have this dirty disease?" She was also presenting with genuine questions of relationship: "Is this contagious? Can my boyfriend get it?"

And small as her problem might be, small as her questions might be, the ultimate term of each of these questions is transcendent. Health care professionals simply subsume it all under the name of the disease, *tinea corporis*, a fungal infection of the skin of the trunk.

But the routine ought never be boring in health care. The mundane is never far from the transcendent in the healing arts. Health care is the care of persons—beings in relationship with the transcendent. Clinicians are privileged to experience persons intimately in a fantastic, rich, multidimensional fashion.

When I saw this patient, I saw what she did not see. I saw a one-centimeter, somewhat hyperpigmented macule with a slightly raised and reddish edge located on her anterior left shin. I saw a dermatophyte infection. She saw "I am dirty." I saw her seeing "I am dirty."

Yet the healing commenced immediately, subtly, in a well-choreographed and well-rehearsed ritual. "No, it's not a parasite. It's a fungus. It's very common. Even people who bathe five times a day can get it" ("No, you are not dirty.").

"We can fix it easily. It will take time, but we're glad you came to see us today because we're catching it rather early. Come back in a month if it's not better" ("You are of value.").

"No, it's not contagious. Your boyfriend need not worry. No one at work need worry" ("Your relationships can be restored to normal. You will not die socially or physically. Not now. Someday, but not now.").

"Take this cream" ("Trust me. Enter into this relationship. You will be restored.").

Ten minutes. Bread-and-butter medicine. As mundane as it comes. But if God was not there, God is nowhere.

## 8.17
## Indigenous religions and medicines I: A Latino/a focus
Eliseo Torres, *Healing with Herbs and Rituals*[20]

*This passage explains two diseases and their remedies as understood by tradi-*
*tional Mexican folk healers known as* curanderos, *whose healing practices*
*combine material and spiritual dimensions.*

### Mal de ojo:

Although this sounds as though it is inflicted through malice, the opposite
is the case. Mal de ojo—the evil eye—comes about through excessive admiration, usually of those too weak to absorb it. Babies are the most frequent
victims, but animals can contract ojo, too. Charms are worn by those susceptible to the evil eye. The most common is an adorned seed resembling a
deer's eye called *ojo de venado*.

Why would admiration cause illness? Some scholars say that it arises
from the belief that a person projects something of himself when he ad-
mires another. If the person receiving the admiration can't handle it, either
because of youth or weakness, illness results.

To counteract the effect of the admiration and guard against mal de ojo,
the admirer must touch the person, animal, or object of his admiration.

The symptoms of ojo are similar to those of colic: irritability, drooping
eyes, fever, headache, and vomiting.

### Susto:

Sometimes susto is translated as loss of spirit or even loss of soul. Occasionally, it is translated as shock, though it shouldn't be confused with the life-
threatening medical condition known as shock. A common definition is
fright, or magical fright.

Receiving bad news can cause susto, as can any bad scare. It is thought
that such a scare can temporarily drive the person's spirit or soul from the
body. Susto has to be treated immediately or it will lead to the much more
serious *susto pasado* or, in Mexico, *susto meco*—an old susto that is much
more difficult to treat and can lead to death.

Weakness is a symptom of susto. Or, as Dolores Latorre describes it in
*Cooking and Curing with Mexican Herbs*, "the victim suddenly feels wobbly,
chilly, shaky, limp, and drowsy, or he may develop a headache accompanied
by nausea." On the other hand, when Ari Kiev describes the symptoms in

*Curanderismo*, he writes that they are "a mixture of anxiety—dyspnea, indigestion, palpitations, and depression—loss of interest in things, irritability, insomnia, and anorexia." Kiev relates one curandero's belief that a susto untreated can lead to heart attack.

**8.18**

**Indigenous religions and medicines II: A Native American focus**

Black Elk, *The Sixth Grandfather*[21]

*This passage describing an indigenous ritual of healing is from the transcript of an interview with Black Elk, a healer and spiritual leader of the Native American Lakota tribe. According to the traditional Lakota belief system, the tribe received the knowledge of healing wounds from grizzly bears. Therefore, the imitation of bears is central to "medicine men's" ritualistic performance.*

As I got ready I noticed that there was someone wounded in a tipi and bear medicine men were treating him. This medicine man's name was Hairy Chin and he had about six [five?] sons with him and they had to take part in the ceremony. I was to take part too. They had to have four [six?] young bears [that is, boys to play the role of bears] to help the medicine man. They asked me to sit down beside the four bears and I knew I was to be used as a young bear to help this man to be cured. Then I thought about my vision and it seemed to raise me off the ground. Maybe this medicine man knew that I had this power, so this is why he brought me over.

   . . .

Then the medicine man sang:

   At the doorway the sacred herbs are rejoicing.

   The wounded man, Rattling Hawk, was shot through the hips and was wounded in the Rosebud fight. It seemed to be an impossibility to heal him. They gave him a holy stick painted red. There were two women with the man on either side. One of them had a cup of water and the other girl had an herb. After this song they presented me with the red stick and the cup of water and I looked into the cup expecting to see something in it like a blue man. It was impossible for the wounded [man] to get up and the chief bear told the girls to give the water and herb to the man and then it came to my mind that someday I will have to perform this myself. Then when they gave the wounded man the stick, he stood up. The two girls led [him] out of the tipi and faced the south. Then all the six bears began to groan like bears and you could see flames coming out—all kinds of colors—and feathers coming out. They did this toward the wounded man. Then after this the man began to walk with this sacred red cane.

When I saw all this happen I thought this was part of the vision and that some day I'd be doing this only it would be greater. This bear medicine man came forward and pulled me toward him. He began to chew an herb and blew it into my mouth and then he threw me down and before I knew it I was standing up on my four haunches like a bear. I made a cry and it was a genuine bear sound and I felt like a bear and wanted to grab someone. We all went out of the tipi then acting like bears. After this the medicine man came out and he looked like a real bear to me—a big bear—and he was fierce too.

### 8.19
### The spiritual and the embodied I: An African American focus
Stephanie Mitchem, "Healing Hearts and Broken Bodies"[22]

*This excerpt from the scholar Stephanie Mitchem's essay shed light on the presence of a complex web of spiritual, political, racial, gendered, and cultural dimensions in African American women's pursuits of healing.*

Healing, in a black women's context, is not just about curing physical ills but necessarily includes healing the past, the present, work, income, family, community, spirit, mind, and emotions. This wider, more integrated view of healing aims for wholeness and originates from a configuration of black culture that defines relationships holistically. Such views are practical, creative, enriching, and life giving. The values inherent in these ideas inform black women's spirituality.

A black woman's spirituality is reflective of African American ways of understanding the world and life. From a black cultural view of life, human existence is not carved into separate compartments of body and soul, sacred and profane. Instead, all the assorted pieces overlap into a cosmos that is understood as integrated and whole: each portion of life is interwoven, interrelated, and interdependent. For instance, an older black woman who had played a significant role in the Civil Rights Movement challenged some black college students: "If you think you pulled your own self up by your bootstraps, forget it. Remember those on whose shoulders you stand." To be aware of those who paid the high price for the seeming success of black Americans today is recognition of the connections between the people of the present and those of past generations. This idea is counter to the self-made American myth, in which an individual can accomplish anything on her or his own merit and effort. But, for black Americans, ancestors of the past are not just distant memories.

Throughout this country's history, with or without the support and recognition of differences, African Americans have continued to focus attention and handle events in culturally specific ways. At the core of these constructions is a view that each human life is interconnected with the other—living and deceased and unborn—as well as with nature and the divine. These relationships have a compelling reality that demands honor and action. To fail to do so constitutes a form of sin that damages the physical and emotional, thereby creating illness. These relationships form the core of healing in these black perspectives.

## 8.20
### The spiritual and the embodied II: Hinduism
Mohandas Gandhi, *An Autobiography; or, The Story of My Experiments with Truth*[23]

*This excerpt is from the* Autobiography *of Mohandas Gandhi (1869–1948), the world-famous leader of the Indian independence movement and a follower of Hinduism, who was reverently referred to as Mahatma (Sanskrit for "great soul"). Gandhi saw dietary and health-care choices as important for cultivating spiritual attitudes of restraint and self-control.*

As the ideals of sacrifice and simplicity were becoming more and more realized, and the religious consciousness was becoming more and more quickened in my daily life, the passion for vegetarianism as a mission went on increasing. I have known only one way of carrying on missionary work, viz., by personal example and discussion with searchers for knowledge.

. . .

Though I have had two serious illnesses in my life, I believe that man has little need to drug himself. 999 cases out of a thousand can be brought round by means of a well-regulated diet, water and earth treatment and similar household remedies. He who runs to the doctor, vaidya or hakim for every little ailment, and swallows all kinds of vegetable and mineral drugs, not only curtails his life, but, by becoming the slave of his body instead of remaining its master, loses self-control, and ceases to be a man.

. . .

It is my firm conviction that man need take no milk at all, beyond the mother's milk that he takes as a baby. His diet should consist of nothing but sunbaked fruits and nuts. He can secure enough nourishment both for the tissues and the nerves from fruits like grapes and nuts like almonds. Restraint of the sexual and other passions becomes easy for a man who lives on such food. My coworkers and I have seen by experience that there is much truth in the Indian proverb that as a man eats, so shall he become.

. . .

I know it is argued that the soul has nothing to do with what one eats or drinks, as the soul neither eats nor drinks; that it is not what you put inside from without, but what you express outwardly from within, that matters. There is, no doubt, some force in this. But rather than examine this reasoning, I shall content myself with merely declaring my firm conviction that, for the seeker who would live in fear of God and who would see Him face to face, restraint in diet both as to quantity and quality is as essential as restraint in thought and speech.

## 8.21
## New directions for religion in health care I
Robert Veatch, *Patient, Heal Thyself*[24]

*The contemporary medical ethicist Robert Veatch suggested reforming American health care by creating medical networks of physicians and patients based on shared values, including religious beliefs. Since participants in such networks would be more likely to have similar worldviews, such institutional arrangements would increase the consideration of patients' beliefs and values in clinical care.*

There might be more hope if the patient were to choose her cadre of well-being experts (lawyers, accountants, physicians, et al.) on the basis of what I will call their "deep" value systems. That way, when unconscious bias and distortion occur, as inevitably they must, they will tip the decision in the direction of the patient's own system.

I say "deep" value system because I want to make clear that I am not referring to a cursory assessment of the professional's personality, demeanor, and short-term tastes; that would hardly suffice. If, however, there were alignments—"value pairings"—based on the most fundamental worldviews of the layperson and professional, then there would be some hope. This probably would mean picking providers on the basis of their religious and/or political affiliations, philosophical and social inclinations, and other deeply penetrating worldviews. To the extent that the provider and patient were of the same mind-set, then there is some reason that the technically competent clinician could guess fairly well what would serve the patient's interest—at least much of the time.

The difficulty in establishing a convergence of deep values cannot be underestimated. Surely, it would not be sufficient, for instance, to pair providers and patients on the basis of their institutional religious affiliations. Not all members of a religious denomination think alike. But there is reason to hope that people can find providers with similar deep value orientations, at least for certain types of medical services.

. . .

Providing an institutional framework for pairing based on deep value convergence in more routine health care may be more difficult, but not impossible. HMOs could be organized by social and religious groups that could formally articulate certain value commitments. A Catholic HMO, like a Catholic hospital, could articulate to potential members not only a set of values pertaining to obstetrical and gynecological issues, but also a framework for deciding which treatments may be omitted because they are too burdensome. A liberal Protestant health-care system would announce a different framework; a libertarian secular system still another. A truly Protestant health-care system, for example, would probably reflect the belief that the layperson is capable of having control over the "text." The medical record, accordingly, would be placed in the patient's hands, just as the Bible was.

## 8.22
### New directions for religion in health care II
James Cates, *Serving the Amish*[25]

*This excerpt from a professional manual offered religious and cultural guidance to health-care workers serving separatist Amish communities. The author*

*followed the Amish custom of referring to community outsiders and their*
*culture as "English."*

Once a patient is admitted to a hospital or is in residence at a health care facility, there are minimal but important culture-specific needs. In general,
there are no dietary restrictions; however, food sharing is an important
nurturing practice, serving as a support during times of stress. Furthermore, many Amish prefer traditional American cuisine and may be less
comfortable with contemporary or exotic choices. Silent prayer is offered
before and often after meals. Although a patient may forego the ritual in
deference to English surroundings, the custom is an important one in the
community. Depending on the specific Amish affiliation, both prayers may
be considered a requirement, but for many the prayer prior to the meal is
the more essential rite.

A patient may be familiar with advance directives. However, without
time to consider, reflect, and talk with family members and possibly with
clergy, patients will choose the option perceived as most consistent with
their beliefs. As a result, the default choice will often be to avoid heroic
measures. (I was asked to transport an Amish bishop to the hospital to visit
his wife, who had been taken there in an emergency. The items he took with
him from his home included her living will.) As is the case with any major
decision, they prefer time to consider the potential ramifications before ar-
riving at a final choice. The Amish accept blood transfusions and organ
transplants. They also give blood, and family members will normally donate
if asked.

As their style of dress indicates, Amish people maintain a high level of
modesty. Nevertheless, they usually remain open to opposite-gender health
care workers. Women wear a hair covering at all times. This is normally a
prayer bonnet, but in more casual circumstances they may substitute a
scarf or shawl. A woman's covering should be removed only as an absolute
necessity, and the reason explained beforehand to both the patient and
any family present. (In the incident described above, one of the items the
bishop's wife had explicitly requested was a white handkerchief. When
we arrived at her room, she immediately used it as a head covering, her
*kapp*, or more formal head covering, having been put away with her street
clothes.)

## NOTES

1. Peter J. Brown, "Religion and Global Health," in Idler, *Religion as a Social Determinant of Public Health*, 285.

2. Livingstone, *Missionary Travels and Researches*, n.p.

3. World Vision, "Practicing Faith," n.p.

4. "Questions Answered," 2.

5. "Beginning of World Wide Revival," 1.

6. Reprinted by permission of the publisher from *Testing Prayer: Science and Healing* by Candy Gunther Brown (Cambridge, MA: Harvard University Press, 2012), 194–96. Copyright © 2012 by the President and Fellows of Harvard College.

7. Gyatso, "Science at the Crossroads," http://www.dalailama.com/messages/buddhism/science-at-the-crossroads. Reprinted by permission of the Mind and Life Institute, Boulder, CO, USA.

8. Eddy, *Science and Health*, 147–62.

9. Copyright © Watch Tower Bible and Tract Society of Pennsylvania, http://www.jw.org/en/bible-teachings/questions/bible-about-blood-transfusion/#?insight[search_id]=0ff1aff1-cf27-4090-bbbd-c5a17e35cd4d&insight[search_result_index]=2.

10. Pope Pius XI, "Casti Connubii." Copyright © Libreria Editrice Vaticana.

11. Sanger, "Birth Control Advances." Copyright © Alexander Sanger, Executor of the Estate of Margaret Sanger. Reprinted with permission.

12. Jürgen Habermas, *The Future of Human Nature* (Cambridge: Polity, 2003), 114–15. Reprinted by permission of Polity Press.

13. Excerpt from page 451 of *The Moral Vision of the New Testament* by Richard B. Hays. Copyright © 1996 by Richard B. Hays. Reprinted by permission of Harper-Collins Publishers.

14. Religious Coalition for Reproductive Choice, *Prayerfully Pro-Choice: Resources for Worship*, 86–87.

15. Ibid., 75–76. Diann L. Neu, DMin, LGSW, is cofounder and codirector of the Women's Alliance for Theology, Ethics and Ritual (WATER) in Silver Spring, MD. www.waterwomensalliance.org, dneu@hers.com.

16. Breck, *Sacred Gift of Life*, 223–25.

17. Eilberg, "Jewish Principles of Care for the Dying," 1.

18. William F. May, *The Physician's Covenant: Images of the Healer in Medical Ethics* (Lexington, KY: Westminster John Knox Press, 2000), 22–24. Reprinted with permission.

19. Daniel P. Sulmasy, OFM, MD, *A Balm for Gilead: Meditations on Spirituality and the Healing Arts*, 11–13. Copyright © 2006 by Georgetown University Press. Reprinted with permission. www.press.georgetown.edu.

20. Torres, *Healing with Herbs and Rituals*, 13–15.

21. Reproduced from *The Sixth Grandfather: Black Elk's Teachings Given to John G. Neihardt*, ed. Raymond J. DeMallie, 178–79, by permission of the University of Nebraska Press. Copyright © 1984 by the University of Nebraska Press. All materials from the interviews and other previously unpublished writings by members of the Neihardt family copyright © 1984 by the John G. Neihardt Trust.

22. Mitchem and Townes, *Faith, Health, and Healing*, 184–85.

23. Gandhi, *Autobiography,* in *Collected Works of Mahatma Gandhi,* 39:213–18. www.gandhiheritageportal.org of the Sabarmati Ashram Preservation and Memorial Trust, Ahmedabad. Reprinted by permission of the Navajivan Trust.

24. Veatch, *Patient, Heal Thyself,* 107–8.

25. James A. Cates, *Serving the Amish: A Cultural Guide for Professionals,* 160–61. Copyright © 2014 Johns Hopkins University Press. Reprinted with permission of Johns Hopkins University Press.

# SELECT BIBLIOGRAPHY

Abdel Haleem, M. A. S., trans. *The Qur'an*. Oxford World's Classics. Oxford: Oxford University Press, 2004.

Aquinas, Thomas. *Summa theologiae: Latin Text and English Translation, Introductions, Notes, Appendices, and Glossaries*. Vol. 40. Edited by T. F. O'Meara and M. J. Duffy. New York: Cambridge University Press, 2006.

Augustine. *The City of God*. Translated by Marcus Dods. New York: Modern Library, 1950.

———. *The Confessions of Saint Augustine*. Translated by E. M. Blaiklock. London: Hodder and Stoughton, 1983.

———. *The Retractations*. Translated by Sister Mary Inez Bogan. Vol. 60 of *The Fathers of the Church*. Washington, DC: Catholic University of America Press, 1968.

Azusa Street Mission. "Beginning of World Wide Revival." *Apostolic Faith* 1.5 (January 1907): 1.

———. "Questions Answered." *Apostolic Faith* 1.11 (October 1907–January 1908): 2.

Baghdādī, ʿAbd al-Laṭīf Ibn Yūsuf al-. *The Physician as a Rebellious Intellectual: The Book of the Two Pieces of Advice*. Translated by N. Peter Joosse. Frankfurt: Peter Lang, 2014.

Barstow, Anne Llewellyn. *Witchcraze: A New History of the European Witch Hunts*. San Francisco, CA: Pandora, 1994.

Behr, Charles Allison, trans. *Aelius Aristides and the Sacred Tales*. Amsterdam: A. M. Hakkert, 1968.

Bock, Barbara. *The Healing Goddess Gula: Towards an Understanding of Ancient Babylonian Medicine*. Leiden: Brill, 2014.

Breck, John. *The Sacred Gift of Life: Orthodox Christianity and Bioethics*. Crestwood, NY: St. Vladimir's Seminary Press, 1998.

Brown, Candy Gunther. *Testing Prayer: Science and Healing*. Cambridge, MA: Harvard University Press, 2012.

Bukhārī, Muḥammad al-. *The Translation of the Meanings of Saḥîh Bukhârî*. Translated by Muhammad Muhsin Khan. Riyadh, Saudi Arabia: Dar-us-Salam, 1997.

Burton, Robert [Democritus Junior]. *The Anatomy of Melancholy*. Edited by Karl Hagen. http://www.gutenberg.org/files/10800/10800-h/10800-h.htm.

Bynum, Caroline Walker. *Fragmentation and Redemption: Essays on Gender and the Human Body in Medieval Religion.* Cambridge, MA: Zone, 1991.

——. *Holy Feast and Holy Fast: The Religious Significance of Food to Medieval Women.* Berkeley: University of California Press, 1987.

Bynum, William F. *History of Medicine: A Very Short Introduction.* Oxford: Oxford University Press, 2008.

Calvin, John. *Commentary on a Harmony of the Evangelists, Matthew, Mark, and Luke.* Translated by William Pringle. Grand Rapids, MI: Baker, 1984.

——. *Institutes of the Christian Religion.* Edited by John T. McNeill, translated by Ford Lewis Battles. Louisville, KY: Westminster John Knox, 2006.

Carlstadt, Andreas Bodenstein von. *The Essential Carlstadt: Fifteen Tracts.* Translated and edited by Edward J. Furcha. Waterloo, ON: Herald Press, 1995.

Cates, James A. *Serving the Amish: A Cultural Guide for Professionals.* Baltimore, MD: Johns Hopkins University Press, 2014.

Cohen, Morris R., and I. E. Drabkin. *A Source Book in Greek Science.* Cambridge, MA: Harvard University Press, 1966.

Dawes, Elizabeth, trans. *Three Byzantine Saints: Contemporary Biographies Translated from the Greek.* Crestwood, NY: St. Vladimir's Seminary Press, 1977.

DeMallie, Raymond J., ed. *The Sixth Grandfather: Black Elk's Teachings Given to John G. Neihardt.* Lincoln: University of Nebraska Press, 1984.

Eatough, Geoffrey. *Fracastoro's Syphilis: Introduction, Text, Translation and Notes.* Arca 12. Liverpool, England: Francis Cairns, 1984.

Ebbell, Bendix, trans. *The Papyrus Ebers: The Greatest Egyptian Medical Document.* Copenhagen: Levin and Munksgaard, 1937.

Eddy, Mary Baker. *Science and Health with Key to the Scriptures.* Boston: Christian Science Publishing Society, 1994.

Edelstein, Emma J., and Ludwig Edelstein. *Asclepius: A Collection and Interpretation of the Testimonies.* 1945. 2 vols. in one. Baltimore, MD: Johns Hopkins University Press, 1998.

Edelstein, Ludwig. *The Hippocratic Oath: Text, Translation, and Interpretation.* Baltimore, MD: The Johns Hopkins Press, 1943.

Eilberg, Amy. "Jewish Principles of Care for the Dying." *Outstretched Arm* [National Center for Jewish Healing] (Winter 2001): 1.

Erasmus, Desiderius. *The Essential Erasmus.* 1964. Edited and translated by John Dolan. New York: Penguin, 1983.

Estes, J. Worth. *The Medical Skills of Ancient Egypt.* Rev. ed. Canton, MA: Science History Publications/USA, 1993.

Eusebius. *The History of the Church from Christ to Constantine.* Translated by G. A. Williamson. Harmondsworth, England: Penguin, 1965.

Farmer, D. H., ed. *The Age of Bede.* Translated by J. F. Webb. 1965. London: Penguin, 1998.

Friedenwald, Harry, trans. "Oath and Prayer of Maimonides." *Bulletin of the Johns Hopkins Hospital* 28 (1917): 260–61. http://guides.library.jhu.edu/c.php?g=202502 &p=1335755.

Galen. *On the Usefulness of the Parts of the Body.* Translated by Margaret Tallmadge May. 2 vols. Ithaca, NY: Cornell University Press, 1968.

Gandhi, Mohandas. *An Autobiography; or, The Story of My Experiments with Truth.* In *The Collected Works of Mahatma Gandhi.* Vol. 39. New Delhi: N.p., 1970. www.gandhi heritageportal.org.

Ghazālī, Abū Ḥāmid al-. *Al-Ghazali's Path to Sufism and His Deliverance from Error [al-Munqidh min al-Dalal].* Translated by R. J. McCarthy. Louisville, KY: Fons Vitae, 2000.

Grant, Frederick C., ed. *Ancient Roman Religion.* New York: Liberal Arts Press, 1957.

——. *Hellenistic Religions: The Age of Syncretism.* New York: Liberal Arts Press, 1953.

Grenfell, B. P., and A. S. Hunt, trans. and eds. *The Oxyrhynchus Papyrus.* Pt. 11. London: Egypt Exploration Fund, 1915.

Gyatso, Tenzin, the Dalai Lama. "Science at the Crossroads." http://www.dalailama .com/messages/buddhism/science-at-the-crossroads.

Habermas, Jürgen. *The Future of Human Nature.* Cambridge: Polity, 2003.

Hajjāj, Muslim Ibn al-. *English Translation of Sahih Muslim.* Translated by Nasiruddin al-Khattab. Ḥadīth edited by Ḥāfiz Abu Ṭāhir Zubair ʿAli Zaʾi and translation edited by Huda Khattab. Riyadh, Saudi Arabia: Dar-us-Salam, 2007.

Harnack, Adolf. *The Mission and Expansion of Christianity in the First Three Centuries.* Translated and edited by James Moffatt. 3 vols. New York: Putnam's, 1904.

Hays, Richard B. *The Moral Vision of the New Testament.* San Francisco, CA: Harper-Collins, 1996.

Hildegard of Bingen. *On Natural Philosophy and Medicine: Selections from Cause et Cure.* Translated by Margaret Berger. Cambridge: D. S. Brewer, 1999.

*Hippocrates.* 4 vols. Translated and edited by W. H. S. Jones. Loeb Classical Library. Cambridge, MA: Harvard University Press, 1923–31.

Homer. *The Iliad.* 1924. Translated by A. T. Murray, revised by William F. Wyatt, edited by Jeffery Henderson. Loeb Classical Library. Cambridge, MA: Harvard University Press, 1999.

Ibn ʿAṭāʾ Allāh al-Iskandarī. *The Key to Salvation: A Sufi Manual of Invocation.* Translated by Mary Ann Koury Danner. Cambridge: Islamic Texts Society, 1996.

Ibn Hindū, Abū al-Faraj ʿAlī Ibn al-Ḥusayn. *Ibn al-Hindu: The Key to Medicine and a Guide for Students.* Translated by Aida Tibi. Reading, England: Garnet, 2011.

Ibn Qayyim al-Jawzīya. *Medicine of the Prophet.* Translated by Penelope Johnstone. Cambridge: Islamic Texts Society, 1998.

Ibn Sīnā, Abū ʿAlī. *al-Kitāb al-Qānūn fī al-Ṭibb* [Arabic]. Būlāq: al-Maṭbaʿah al-ʿĀmirah, 1878. Excerpt translated by M. A. Mujeeb Khan as "On the Definition of Medicine," *Canon of Medicine* (this volume).

Idler, Ellen L., ed. *Religion as a Social Determinant of Public Health.* New York: Oxford University Press, 2014.

Ignatius of Loyola. *Ignatius of Loyola: The Spiritual Exercises and Selected Works.* Edited by George E. Ganss. New York: Paulist Press, 1991.

——. *The Spiritual Exercises of St. Ignatius of Loyola.* Translated by Charles Seager. London: Charles Dolman, 1847.

Josephus. *Jewish Antiquities: Books VII–VIII.* 1934. Translated by Ralph Marcus, edited by G. P. Goold. Loeb Classical Library. Cambridge, MA: Harvard University Press, 1998.

Julian. *The Works of Emperor Julian.* Vol. 3. Translated by Emily Wilmer Cave Wright. Loeb Classical Library. Cambridge, MA: Harvard University Press, 1913.

Julian of Norwich. *Showings.* Translated by Edmund Colledge and James Walsh. New York: Paulist Press, 1978.

King, E. J. *The Rule, Statutes, and Customs of the Hospitallers, 1099–1310.* New York: AMC Press, 1980.

Lee, T'ao. "Medical Ethics in Ancient China." *Bulletin of the History of Medicine* 13 (1943): 268–77.

Lewis, Naphtali, and Meyer Reinhold, eds. *Roman Civilization: Sourcebook I: The Republic.* 1951. New York: Harper and Row, 1966.

Lichtheim, Miriam. *Ancient Egyptian Literature: A Book of Readings,* vol. 3: *The Late Period.* Berkeley: University of California Press, 1980.

Livingstone, David. *Missionary Travels and Researches in South Africa.* London: John Murray, 1857. http://www.gutenberg.org/files/1039/1039-h/1039-h.htm.

Livy. *Livy, in Fourteen Volumes.* Vol. 3 (Books 5, 6, 7). Translated by B. O. Foster. 1924. Loeb Classical Library. Cambridge, MA: Harvard University Press, 1984.

Lloyd, Geoffrey E. R. *In the Grip of Disease: Studies in the Greek Imagination.* Oxford: Oxford University Press, 2003.

Luck, Georg, ed. and trans. *Arcana Mundi: Magic and the Occult in the Greek and Roman Worlds: A Collection of Ancient Texts.* 2nd ed. Baltimore, MD: Johns Hopkins University Press, 2006.

Luther, Martin. *The Babylonian Captivity of the Church.* In *Works of Martin Luther with Introductions and Notes.* Philadelphia: A. J. Holman, 1915. Translated by Albert T. W. Steinhaeuser, edited and modernized by Robert E. Smith (last modified December 3, 2002). http://www.projectwittenberg.org/etext/luther/babylonian /babylonian.htm#8.

———. *Luther's Works, American Edition.* 55 vols. Edited by J. Pelikan and H. T. Lehmann. St. Louis, MO: Concordia, and Philadelphia: Fortress, 1955–86.

Mackay, Christopher S., trans. *The Hammer of Witches: A Complete Translation of the Malleus Maleficarum.* New York: Cambridge University Press, 2009.

Maimonides, Moses. *Ethical Writings of Maimonides.* Edited by Raymond Weiss and Charles Butterworth. New York: New York University Press, 1975.

Majūsī, ʿAlī Ibn al-ʿAbbās al-. "Kitāb Kāmil al-Ṣināʿa fī al-Ṭibb." Arabic MS 4, Cushing/ Whitney Medical Library, Yale University. Translated by M. A. Mujeeb Khan as "Complete Book on the Art of Medicine" (this volume).

May, William F. *The Physician's Covenant: Images of the Healer in Medical Ethics.* Lexington, KY: Westminster John Knox, 2000.

Miller, Timothy S., and John W. Nesbitt. *Walking Corpses: Leprosy in Byzantium and the Medieval West.* Ithaca, NY: Cornell University Press, 2014.

Mitchem, Stephanie Y., and Emilie Maureen Townes, eds. *Faith, Health, and Healing in African American Life.* Westport, CT: Praeger, 2008.

Nock, A. D. *Conversion: The Old and the New in Religion from Alexander the Great to Augustine of Hippo.* London: Oxford University Press, 1933.

Origen. *Contra Celsum.* 1953. Translated by Henry Chadwick. Cambridge: Cambridge University Press, 1980.

Paracelsus. *The Hermetic and Alchemical Writings of Aureolus Philippus Theophrastus Bombast, Called Paracelsus the Great.* Translated by Arthur Edward Waite. London: J. Elliott, 1894.

Paré, Ambroise. *Journeys in Diverse Places.* Translated by Stephen A. Paget. Hoboken, NJ: Generic NL Freebook Publisher, eBook Collection (EBSCOhost), 1990.

Peet, T. Eric, trans. *A Comparative Study of the Literatures of Egypt, Palestine, and Mesopotamia: Egypt's Contribution to the Literatures of the Ancient World.* 1931. Eugene, OR: Wipf and Stock, 2007.

Pierozzi, Antoninus. "The Diverse Vices of Physicians and Their Salaries." In *Medieval Medicine: A Reader.* Edited by Faith Wallis. Toronto: University of Toronto Press, 2010.

Pius XI. "Casti Connubii." 1930. https://w2.vatican.va/content/pius-xi/en/encyclicals/documents/hf_p-xi_enc_19301231_casti-connubii.html.

Pliny. *Natural History.* Vol. 8. Translated by W. H. S. Jones. Loeb Classical Library. Cambridge, MA: Harvard University Press, 1963.

Plutarch. *Life of Cato the Elder.* In *The Makers of Rome: Plutarch.* Translated by Ian Scott-Kilvert. London: Penguin Classics, 1965.

Porterfield, Amanda. *Healing in the History of Christianity.* New York: Oxford University Press, 2005.

Pritchard, James B., ed. *Ancient Near Eastern Texts Relating to the Old Testament.* 2nd ed. Princeton, NJ: Princeton University Press, 1955.

Raymond of Capua. *The Life of St. Catherine of Siena.* Translated by George Lamb. London: Harvill, 1960.

Rāzī, Abū Bakr Zakarīyā al-. *Kitāb manāfiʿ al-aghdhiya wa dafʿ maḍārrihā* [Arabic]. Miṣr: al-Maṭbaʿa al-Khayrīya, 1884. Translated by M. A. Mujeeb Khan as "On the Benefits of Nutrition and Dispelling Its Harms" (this volume).

Religious Coalition for Reproductive Choice. *Prayerfully Pro-Choice: Resources for Worship.* N.p.: Religious Coalition for Reproductive Choice, 2004.

Roberts, A., and J. Donaldson, eds. *The Ante-Nicene Fathers.* Vols. 3 and 4. Edinburgh: Clark, 1866–1872. Available at http://www.tertullian.org/anf/index.htm.

Ruhāwī, Isḥāq Ibn ʿAlī al-. *Ethics of the Physician.* Translated by Martin Levey. In Martin Levey, "Medical Ethics of Medieval Islam with Special Reference to al-Ruhāwī's 'Practical Ethics of the Physician.'" *Transactions of the American Philosophical Society* 57.3 (1967): 1–100.

Sanger, Margaret. "Birth Control Advances: A Reply to the Pope" (1931). Margaret Sanger Papers, Sophia Smith Collection, Smith College, Margaret Sanger Microfilm, S71:243. http://www.nyu.edu/projects/sanger/webedition/app/documents/show.php?sangerDoc=236637.xml.

Schaff, Philip, and Henry Wace, eds. *Nicene and Post-Nicene Fathers.* Edinburgh: Clark, n.d. Available at http://www.ccel.org/fathers.html.

Scurlock, JoAnn. *Sourcebook for Ancient Mesopotamian Medicine.* Atlanta, GA: SBL Press, 2014.

Suetonius. *Lives of the Caesars.* 2 vols. Translated by J. C. Rolf. Loeb Classical Library. Cambridge, MA: Harvard University Press, 1914.

Sulmasy, Daniel P. *A Balm for Gilead: Meditations on Spirituality and the Healing Arts.* Washington, DC: Georgetown University Press, 2006.

Suyūṭī, ʿAbd al-Raḥmān Jalāl al-Dīn al-. *As-Suyuti's* Tibb an-Nabbi: *Medicine of the Prophet.* 1994. Edited by Ahmad Thompson, adapted from a translation by Cyril Elgood. London: Ta-Ha, 2015.

Tanner, Norman P. *Decrees of the Ecumenical Councils.* Washington, DC: Georgetown University Press, 1990.

Teresa of Ávila. *The Interior Castle.* 1577. Translated by Kieran Kavanaugh and Otilio Rodriguez. New York: Paulist Press, 1979.

Thucydides. *History of the Peloponnesian War.* 1954. Translated by Rex Warner. London: Penguin, 1972.

Thurston, Robert W. *Witch, Wicce, Mother Goose: The Rise and Fall of the Witch Hunts in Europe and North America.* Edinburgh: Longman, 2001,

Torres, Eliseo. *Healing with Herbs and Rituals: A Mexican Tradition.* Edited by Timothy Leighton Sawyer. Albuquerque: University of New Mexico Press, 2006.

Veatch, Robert M. *Patient, Heal Thyself: How the New Medicine Puts the Patient in Charge.* New York: Oxford University Press, 2009.

Wallis, Faith, ed. *Medieval Medicine: A Reader.* Toronto: University of Toronto Press, 2010.

Watch Tower Bible and Tract Society of Pennsylvania. "What Does the Bible Say About Blood Transfusions?" http://www.jw.org/en/bible-teachings/questions/bible-about -blood-transfusion/#?insight[search_id]=0ff1aff1-cf27-4090-bbbd-c5a17e35cd4d &insight[search_result_index]=2.

Wesley, John. *Primitive Physick; or, An Easy and Natural Method of Curing Most Diseases.* Edinburgh: Thornton and Collie, 1846.

White, Carolinne, ed. and trans. *Early Christian Lives.* London: Penguin, 1998.

——. *The Rule of Benedict.* London: Penguin, 2008.

World Vision. "Practicing Faith." http://www.worldvision.org/our-impact/our-faith-in -action.

# INDEX

Aaron, 23, 25

Abbasids, 163, 164–65

abortion, 62, 63, 64, 186, 226–27, 244–46.
See also childbirth

Abū Bakr al-Ṣiddīq, 162

Abu'd-Darda, 186

Achilles, 43, 44, 45

Adam and Eve, 136, 150, 191, 243. See also Fall

Aelfflaed, 140

Aelius Aristides, 72; Sacred Tales, 84–88

African Americans, 228, 255–56

Agamemnon, 43, 44, 46

Agdistis, shrine of, 64

alchemy, 192, 205

Alexander the Great, 1, 28, 42

Alexandria, 102

'Alī Ibn Abī Ṭālib, 162

Alypius, 119

Ambrose, 103, 119

Ambrosia, 65, 66

Amish, 228, 258–59

amulets, 2, 3, 43, 72, 89, 103. See also magic

Anabaptists, 190, 200

anarieis (impotence), 50–52

animism, 70, 74

anointing, 101, 108–9

Anthony, 103, 121–22

Antoninus Pierozzi, Summa theologica moralis, 137–38

Antu, 9

Anu, 8, 9

Anunītum, 9

Apollo, 39, 43, 44–45, 47, 57, 63, 75, 237

Apollonius of Tyana, 73, 94–95

Apostolic Constitution, 102

Aquinas, Thomas, Summa theologiae, 137, 152–53

Arabs, 163, 165–66

Archagathus, 71, 77, 78

Aristotle, 81, 175–76; The Book of Dialectics, 176

asceticism, 94, 117, 122, 132, 134, 135, 148–49, 189, 193

Asklepios (Asclepius, Aesculapius), 21, 65–67, 68, 73, 84–89, 111, 208; and Epidaurus, 41–42, 64, 65, 71, 72, 77; and Eusebius, 89–90; and Hippocratic Oath, 63; and Pergamum, 41, 72, 84, 88–89

astrology, 72, 73, 97–98. See also cosmos/ universe

Athanasius, Life of Anthony, 121–22

Athens, 41, 48, 57–62

Augustine, 137, 151, 153, 241, 242; The City of God, 74–75, 103–4, 119–21, 152, 153; Confessions, 118–19; De bono coniugali, 239; De doctrina Christiana, 152; de Vera religione, 118; Retractations, 118

Avicenna. See Ibn Sīnā, Abū 'Alī (Avicenna)

Azusa Street Mission, Apostolic Faith, 232–33

Azusa Street revival, 223–24

Babylon, 1, 2, 4, 11, 92, 95

al-Baghdādī, 'Abd al-Laṭīf Ibn Yūsuf, 165; The Book of the Two Pieces of Advice, 180–81

Baker, Heidi, 233–35

Basileias, 103, 125–26

Basil the Great, 103, 122, 125–26